LIGHT

HEALTH BENEFITS & MEDICAL APPLICATIONS

Discover How Light Heals

MATT DEBOW

EDITOR
Dan Terry

CITATIONS
Kenneth Myers, Ph.D.

GLOSSARY
Rim Schreiber

Book Formatting
Dan Terry and Ben Lennon

RESEARCH, DEVELOPMENT & ACQUISITIONS
Manuel Inverno, Brian Hulbert, Bill Levinson, Ph.D., Diva Seddick, M.D., Miles Newcombe, Charles Oliphant, Hurley Young, Jeanne M. Fahey, Alexander Radaev, Ph.D., Jacob Davis and Victor Ho.

EDITORIAL ASSISTANCE & CONSULTANTS
Siobhan Welch, Hope Malkan, Liz & Michael Bensinger, Claudia Zanolini, Patricia DeBow, Pat Smith, Janis Bookout, Stacy Booth, Elizabeth Nakahara, Teresa Seale, Yara Munck, Taryn Chavez, Nirmala Nataraj, Kristin Cerda and Allyson Whipple.

TECHNICAL AND SCIENTIFIC ACKNOWLEDGEMENTS
Eugene Barnett, David Olszewski, E.E., I.E., Bill Levinson, Ph.D., and Kurt Wedgely.

THANKS & DEDICATION
To the people I interviewed for this book and documentary, and individuals who educate others about important health and medical breakthroughs.

INSPIRATIONAL ACKNOWLEDGEMENTS
Michael Shuster, Michelle Nassopoulos, Sandra DeBow, Len Saputo, M.D., Joaquin Carr, Tommy Perez, Kirsten Miller, Mark Commerford, Brian Whaley, Mike Somers, Raleigh DeBow, Georgia Brauer, Brian Leonard, Boris Zemelman, Ph.D., Bob Distefano, Mary Cummins, Nathan Bryan, Ph.D., Kevin Criqui, Susan Bostwick, Bernie Silverman, Jim Thompson, Brooke Luciano, and Seth Ashby.

PERSONAL THANKS
Fred Kahn, M.D., Dr. Bill Levinson, Ph.D., Dr. Ronald Hsu, M.D., Wolfgang Neuberger, Ph.D. and John Strisower.

VERY SPECIAL THANKS

LuxWaves Inc., Medical Light Association, Meditech International, Biolitec AG, University of Texas, Neogenis Inc., Photonics West, International Photodynamic Association, Health Medicine Institute, Light Energy Co., Alpha Spectrum Inc., Stanford University, MedX, U.C. Davis Medical Center, Sutter Medical Center, WCSAR, NASA, Cerus Corporation, Innerg Herbals, VisionScape Studios, Solta Medical Inc., Long Beach Medical Center, Health & Wellness Foundation, Thor International, Harris Medical Resources, and Harvard Medical School.

THANKS TO

Millennium Dental Technologies, Inc., Quantum Devices, Inc., Medtronic, Cyberkinetics Neurotechnology Systems, Inc., NuvoLase Inc, L'Oreal, Avon, Proctor & Gamble, Johnson & Johnson, Palomar, Syneron Medical Ltd., Ageless Beauty, Pharos Life, Neutrogena, L'Oreal, Light BioScience LLC., Solta Medical, My Skincare Boutique, Anodyne Therapy LLC., Laser & Skin Surgery Center of Northern California, Laser & Skin Surgery Center of New York and Cynosure Inc.

Laureen

LIGHT:
Health Benefits & Medical Applications

Published by
Matt DeBow

ISBN 978-0-9845469-0-9

www.MattDeBow.com

10/16

Dedication

To my family's oldest, newest and past members

Table of Contents

DISCLOSURE/GENERAL DISCLAIMER

This book is intended to educate and not to provide medical advice or professional services. The information provided should not be used for diagnosing or treating a health problem or disease; it is not a substitute for professional care. If you have or suspect you may have a health problem, you should consult your health care professional.

The transcription, content development and editorial help were a necessary process, but translation loss in some incidences is inevitable. Transforming medical, scientific and technical information into understandable terms was not an easy process. Since I am not a doctor, scientist or physicists the translation might be incorrect, slightly skewed or misinterpreted.

From within or from behind, a light shines
through us upon things, and makes us aware
that we are nothing, but the light is all.

Ralph Waldo Emerson
1803–1882

INTRODUCTION

En•**light**•en to give knowledge or truth to; endow with spiritual understanding; to free from ignorance, prejudice, or superstition, to make clear the facts or nature of something; inform; illuminate; truth.

Light is part of our physiological make-up, and all living things are photobiological beings. Light is now known to be a part of our cellular biological communication. Technology is allowing us to speak the language of light with living cells.

The body is a "living photocell," stimulated and regulated by light entering our eyes and penetrating the skin. The human photoreceptor molecules are not limited to the retina but are found virtually in all tissue.

Light has the potential to revolutionize medicine in much same the way vaccines and antibiotics have. This book contains information the large pharmaceutical companies don't want you to know, like how light technologies are often more effective than traditional medicine, cost less money and have virtually no side effects. Drug-free treatments are the way of the future and light technology is the conduit by which we'll get there.

The substantial growth in alternative and naturopathic treatment clearly reflects a new trend in medicine. During the course of my research for the documentary and this book, I came across several success stories of people healing with light. I met individuals who had been treated for cancer, debilitating pain, non-healing wounds, injuries and inflammation. For all of them, light had been their only salvation. Some patients had been unable to function normally and the damage was so severe even doctors had given up hope. Once these patients found the light, they were healed beyond anyone's beliefs; in many cases, even their own.

What surprised me most were the accounts of beneficial secondary effects caused by biostimulation light therapy. Finding positive side effects from medical treatments was surprising, and as I interviewed people and sifted through data, I began to understand how this was possible. On my journey I visited Dr. Fred Kahn a leader in the field of photobiological therapy, and spoke with many of his patients. In one case, a patient has been in a serious road accident and was unable to walk without using two canes. This guy had tried every conventional and alternative therapy, but with no success. After beginning light therapy at one of Kahn clinics, it was just a short time before the patient experienced less pain and increased mobility, and eventually, he was able to freely walk again without the walking sticks. In fact, knowing him afterwards made it difficult for me to even imagine him in his previous condition.

Some of Kahn's favorite patients are the skeptics because he knows there is no placebo effect. One skeptic was a well-respected doctor and medical writer who happened to be Kahn's neighbor. When this man's back went out, he arrived at Kahn's clinic laid out flat in the back of a van. Soon, Kahn came to the rescue. After a handful of treatments over a short period of time, the patient was back on his feet. Astounded by his own rapid recovery, he wrote a great story featuring Meditech International, Kahn and his team. Kahn's medical equipment is now used by professional athletes and medical professional all over the world.

In summary, the possibilities for medical light technologies are endless and are being used today for speedy injury recovery, sciatica, non-healing wounds, spinal cord injury, cancer, blood infections, HIV, brain stimulation, Alzheimer's disease, diabetic lesions, cosmetics, dentistry, pain management, fungus eradication, seasonal affective order, and more.

It's important to note that these technologies do not just offer symptomatic relief; light actually cures ailments and disease without masking the problem or drowning it in toxic drugs that could potentially harm the human body. Instead, the spectrum of light used in photobiological treatments spans the rainbow, from ultraviolet to infrared, to select wavelengths in-between. These systems hold the keys to open doors to better health, as you will see. Breakthrough technology in medicine has arrived, now the choice is before us.

Matt DeBow
Austin, Texas
2012

PREFACE

My interest in health and wellness began when I was just a child watching the next door neighbor make liquid from a machine that looked about as strange as "carrot juice" sounded back then. But what really struck me was how she kept her cancer-stricken husband alive for so many years, despite his doctors' predictions. That memory has stayed with me, and the impact has turned out to be life-changing in stimulating my curiosity about health and motivating my quest for alternative therapies. For decades I have searched bookstores and health food stores, attended seminars, presentations and conventions, collecting information about maintaining good health.

Several things I came across were shocking. When I learned food chemicals are found in nearly all processed food products and a daily American diet includes several hundred milligrams of these toxins, I was dumbfounded. Several years later while attending the State of the World Forum convention, a speaker discussing environmental toxicity and its effect on children caught my interest. The major toxin contributor? Food, of course! The term used to describe it was "TILT" (Toxic Induced Loss of Tolerance), resulting in negative health effects and problematic brain functions in children caused by manmade chemicals. This particular speaker pointed out that TILT was the underlying cause of several diseases and long-term health issues.

I began investigating therapies that show promise. Surprisingly, I discovered magnets have been used to promote good health for 3000 years and are still used today by some professional athletes for pain management. There has also been success breaking up kidney stones using of audio shock waves. Another interesting technology uses radio frequencies focused to break apart viruses or bacteria, the same way glass can shatter from exposure to a sound wave of the specific resonant frequency inherent in the chemical composition of the glass.

But what really caught my interest were the studies on light. I learned that some doctors were having great success treating cancer and other diseases and ailments with light, so I published an article called "Electromagnetic Healing; Using Light, Radio Waves, Magnetics & Sound Vibration to Heal the Body and Kill Viruses" that focused on several non-traditional or alternative ways to heal the body, known in the industry as complementary and alternative medicine (CAM). As my research progressed, I eventually produced the documentary *Healing with Light: Advanced Medical Technology* in 2001 on the applications of light in medicine.

Since then, the use of light in medicine has grown exponentially. Drawing on years of research, I have condensed the information into this book to enlighten people, as well as motivate medical professionals to look into these new photobiological technologies. I believe the use of light has the potential to change health care, and ultimately, the way we live.

Chapter One: The History of Light Therapy

Therapy using light radiation is not a new phenomenon. Healing with light began with ancient cultures that revered the sun as a deity and knew light was an effective remedy for illness. Today, the use of light in healing has evolved into several treatments including photodynamic therapy, biostimulation and blood irradiation.

ANCIENT BELIEFS ABOUT LIGHT

Ancient Egyptian healers recognized that certain colors cured mental and physical ailments. Certain Egyptian buildings were constructed, some believe, so that when sunlight entered the temple, its rays split into the colors of the spectrum. These individual colors were directed into different rooms to bathe patients in the color that their state of health required.[1]

The Atharva Veda, a sacred Indian text written in 1400 B.C., mentions using seed extracts as a sunlight activation agent. Other ancient Sanskrit writings describe the body's seven major energy centers or "chakras." Each chakra is considered a source of spiritual energy activated by different colors of the light spectrum, thus affecting our health and well being. This early concept is the first recorded belief that the human body emanates light.[2]

Awareness of the use of light for healing purposes is also reflected in ancient Greek mythology, with the name Orpheus meaning "one who heals with light."[3] People practiced heliotherapy, whole-body exposure to sunlight for health restoration in ancient Greece. Heliotherapy is derived from the Greek word "heliopolis," meaning "city of the sun." Herodotus, the father of heliotherapy, was the first Greek to document both the theory and the practice of solar therapy.[4]

The Greek philosopher Pythagoras used color therapy, and Grecian theorists believed that light shining through the eyes was the most accessible path to the body's internal organs.[5] In 300 B.C. Euclid wrote *Optica* in which

---

[1] Hunt, Roland. "Fragrant & Radiant Healing Symphony." (1999)
[2] Bloomfield, M. The Atharvaveda. (2008)
[3] Schure, Edouard. The Great Initiates. Part 1. (1889)
[4] Liberman, Jacob, Light: Medicine of the Future - How We Can Use It to Heal Ourselves. (1993)
[5] Clark, Linda A. The Ancient Art of Color Therapy. (1975)

he studied the properties of light. He mathematically analyzed light and concluded it traveled in straight lines and was able to describe the laws of reflection.[6]

Around the first century B.C., the *Vishnu Purana* refers to sunlight as "the seven rays of the sun."[7] During the same time period, Greek physician Aurelius Celsus believed specific colors could be used for healing specific ailments.[8] In 125 A.D., Apuleius experimented with flickering light and epilepsy.[9] Centuries later, Islamo-Aristotelian physician Avicenna published *Canon of Medicine* in 1025, emphasizing the importance of color in treating illness.[10]

The simplicity of using light to heal seems too good to be true. As with other naturopathic therapeutic fields like homeopathy, acupuncture and hypnosis, light therapy has encountered a general reluctance in Western medicine to legitimize the field. Western medicine is built upon research, and funding that is largely earmarked for more "legitimate" areas of study. As a result, the field of light therapy is a mixed bag of fringe researchers, independent practitioners, medical specialists, developers and more recently, the United States Government.

Considering the lengthy history of light therapy and its uses all over the world, there is huge potential for improving society's overall health, providing low-cost healing and preventative therapies, diagnosing diseases and ailments and who knows what else?

EARLY SCIENTIFIC BREAKTHROUGHS IN LIGHT

. In the late 1700's, scientists studied the influence of sunlight on human growth and the effects of sunlight deprivation. In 1797 in *The Art of Prolonging Human Life*, Christoph Wilhelm Hufeland writes about the influence of sunlight on human growth, observing that human beings become pale, flabby and apathetic as a result of light deprivation, and eventually lose all vital energy.[11]

---

[6] Euclid. Optica.
[7] Wilson, H. H. The Vishnu Paruna. (2009)
[8] River, C. De Medicina. (2011)
[9] Jeavons, P. and Harding, G. Photosenstive Epilepsy: A Review of the Literature and a Study of 460 Patients. (1975)
[10] Bakhtiar, L. The Canon of Medicine. (1999)
[11] Hufeland, Chritoph Wilhelm. The Art of Prolonging Human Life. (1797)

In the 1870s James Clerk Maxwell published several books detailing mathematical descriptions of magnetic fields He concluded light was a form of electromagnetic radiation. [12] Around the same period, Heinrich Hertz, using Maxwell's theories, successfully generated and detected radio waves in his laboratory and demonstrated that these waves behaved similar to visible light. Hertz's experiments led directly to the development of radio, television, radar, imaging, and wireless communications. [13]   His name is used in measuring pulse rates units, cycles per second (Hz), like in computer speeds (Gigahertz).

At the turn of the 19th century, sunlight was widely used as an antibacterial agent to disinfect operating rooms, as well as to treat wounds, burns, and respiratory infections.[14] General Augustus J. Pleasanton discovered that grapes harvested in a green house with blue transparent windowpanes grew larger. Pleasanton also found that blue light cured certain diseases, affected fertility and stimulated glands. His insights led to the discovery that rays of light toward the violet end of the spectrum (UV) kill bacteria. [15]

During the turn of the century, the world's leading scientists developed theories that would have a tremendous impact on the field of photobiology (the study of the effects of light on living organisms). In 1893 Danish physician Neils Finsen discovered that red light could heal skin disorders such as small pox lesions.[16] Finsen developed a device using a carbon arc filtered through a quartz prism that produced positive results in healing his patients. In 1896 the Finsen Institute was founded in Copenhagen and international recognition won Finsen a Nobel Prize in 1903. Today, Finsen is considered the father of photobiology.

In 1900 Max Planck developed a theory based on light and electromagnetic radiation. His theory largely involved particles of light he named "photons."[17] The scientific community finally agreed that light was a wave, and the original particle theory was gone until Albert Einstein shocked the world in 1905 and said it was both waves and particles.[18] His ideas were

---

[12] Maxwell, J. C.A Treatise on Electricity and Magnetism. (1873)
[13] Hertz, H. Electric Waves. (1893)
[14] Kime, Zane R. Sunlight. (1980)
[15] Pleasonton, A. J. The Influence of the Blue Ray of the Sunlight and the Blue Color of the Sky. (1856)
[16] Finsen, N. R. Om Lysets Indvirkninger paa Huden. (1893)
[17] Tipler, P. A. Modern Physics. (1978)
[18] Einstein, A. Über einen die Erzeugung und Verwandlung des Lichtes betreffenden heuristischen Gesichtspunkt. (1905)

met initially with skepticism among established physicists. But eventually the wave-particle duality light explanation and photoelectric effect would triumph. By then Einstein had received the Nobel Prize in 1921 for his work. Also in the 1920s, Russians discovered ultra-weak photon emissions radiating from living tissues.[19]

The actions, mechanisms and therapeutic value of light began to pique scientists' interest. While Plank, Einstein and Gurwitsch were making advances in physics, other scientists were publishing studies on the medical applications of light. These pioneers include A. Osborne Eaves,[20] Margaret Abigail Cleaves,[21] Hugo Bach[22] and Percy Hall.[23]

The idea that a lack of specific light wavelengths causes biochemical and hormonal deficiencies in both plant and animal cells was conceived by Dr. Wendell Krieg in 1932, Professor of Anatomy at Northwestern University. According to Krieg, these were examples of a condition he called "malillumination."[24]

In 1942 Russian scientist S.V. Krakov discovered that the color red stimulates the sympathetic portion of the autonomic nervous system, while blue stimulates the parasympathetic portion. These findings were later confirmed by researcher Robert Gerard in 1958.[25] Gerard's studies showed that red light increases blood pressure, while blue and white light decrease it. In the same year, Professor and photobiologist Dr. Harry Wohlfarth noticed similar results with a wider range of color wavelengths. During the 1950s, studies found sunlight alleviated neonatal jaundice. By accident Dr. Richard Cremer of United Kingdom discovered jaundiced babies overcame their health problems when in nurseries flooded with blue light.[26] Dr. Max Luscher found an individual's preference for one color and a dislike for

---

[19] A.G. Gurwitsch, S. Grabje and S. Salkind, Die Natur des spezifischen Erregers der Zellteilung. (1923)
[20] Eaves, A. Osborne, The Colour Cure. (1901)
[21] Cleaves, Margaret Abigail, Light Energy: It's Physics, Physiological Action and Therapeutic Applications. (1904)
[22] Bach, Hugo, Ultra-Violet Light by Means of the Alpine Sun Lamp, Treatment and Indications. (1916)
[23] Hall, Percy, Ultra-Violet Rays in the Treatment and Cure of Disease. (1928)
[24] Krieg, Wendell J.S. "The Hypothalamus of the Albino Rat" The Journal of Comparative Neurology, Vol. 55, Issue 1. (1932)
[25] Gerard, R. Differential effects of colored lights on psychophysiological functions. (1958)
[26] Cremer, R. J., Perryman, P.W., Richards, D. H. Influence of light on the hyperbilirubinemia of infants. (1958)

another had a definite meaning that perhaps reflected a pre-existing state of mind, glandular imbalance or both.[27]

Therapeutic light research continued throughout the 1960's when it was discovered that tumors in laboratory mice were affected by specific wavelengths of light. An article written in 1963 by John Ott, inventor of time-lapse photography and the full spectrum light bulb, his research was published in an American Medical Association (AMA) news release to the *Chicago Tribune*.[28] Ott's preliminary research showed lab animals with fast-acting tumors lived only twenty-nine days under cool white florescent light, while their counterparts lived forty-three days under natural sunlight.

The first successful laser treatment (light amplification by stimulated emission of radiation) was developed at Hughes Research Laboratories, and its inventor Charles Townes received the Nobel Prize in 1964. By 1967 Hungarian physician Dr. Andre Mester was performing a series of experiments on animals in an attempt to destroy cancer with lasers. The effort was unsuccessful. To Mester's surprise, the tumor cells were not destroyed. He noticed, however, that the incision where he had implanted the tumors healed extremely quickly. [29] He also noticed that the shaven hair grew faster on the treated group than the untreated group. Because of this work, Mester is considered the father of biostimulation and is credited with discovering the positive biological effects of low power lasers.[30] By the 1970s he was successfully using lasers to treat patients suffering from skin ulcers, burns and infectious wounds.

Another important discovery in the late sixties involves light when it enters the eyes. Light entering the eye causes nerve impulses that influence the lower brain and pituitary gland and trigger the release of hormones. Dr. Joseph Meites of Michigan State University states, "We have no idea how many diseases are linked to hormonal problems, but we do know that several diseases such as diabetes, infertility, cancer and thyroid disorders are involved with hormonal imbalances."[31]

Theoretical biophysicist Fritz-Albert Popp and his research group at the University of Marburg, Germany published a groundbreaking article in

---

[27] Lüscher, M. The Lüscher Colour Test: Remarkable Test That Reveals Your Personality Through Color. (1972)
[28] Ott, John. "The Effects of Natural and Artificial Light on Man and Other Living Things" Chicago Tribune. (1963)
[29] Mester, E., Szende, B., and Tota, J.G. Effect of laser on hair growth of mice. (1967)
[30] Perera, J. The 'healing laser' comes into the limelight. (1987)
[31] Meites, J. The Investigation of Hypothalamic-Pituitary-Adrenal Function. (1969)

1970 about cells emanating light. Popp hypothesized that biophotic action emanating from living tissue is part of a cellular communication system.[32] A few years later, a doctor in New York used a photosensitive drug in combination with a light source to destroy cancer. In 1972 Thomas Dougherty M.D. called this particular process "photodynamic therapy" at Roswell Park Memorial Institute.[33]

In 1979, V. Berezin and K. Martinek found that certain colors of light stimulate specific body enzymes, resulting in five hundred percent greater efficacy, while other colors deactivate certain enzymes and affect the movement of substances across cell membranes. These findings established light as one of the body's prime photobiological regulatory agents.[34]

As a result, light research and technology boomed in the 1980s. In Alberta, Canada, scientist Dr. Harry Woohfarth conducted experiments to evaluate the effects of light and color in educational settings.[35] After painting walls different colors and installing full spectrum lighting, he found that students' academic achievement improved in yellow and orange rooms. Woohfarth also discovered students' blood pressure dropped an average of twenty percent, and interestingly, blind students were also affected.

Also during the 1980s, the National Institute of Mental Health published that seasonal affective disorder (SAD) or "winter depression" could be alleviated by treatment with full spectrum light.[36] In the beginning of the 21st century, the American Cancer Society website published promising data pertaining to several medical light treatments, including photodynamic therapy, biostimulation and blood irradiation.

Today the photobiological effects of light are still being studied and practiced around the world. Although modern Western medicine mainly uses pharmaceuticals to treat illness and disease, light therapy is an emerging technology that can provide affordable alternatives without side effects. With enough public support, light therapy could become a staple of the modern medical community.

---

[32] Rattemeyer, M., Popp, F.A., Nagl, W.: Evidence of photon emission from DNA in living systems. Naturwissenschaften, Vol.68, Nr.11 (1981)

[33] Dougherty, T. J., Henderson, B. W. Photodynamic therapy: basic principles and clinical applications. (1992)

[34] Berezin, I.V., Klyosov, A.A., Martinek, K. General Principles of Enzymatic Catalysis. (1979)

[35] Whlfarth, H. Color and light effects on student's achievement, behavior and physiology. (Edmonton, Atlanta 1986)

[36] Rosenthal, Norman. Seasonal Affective Disorder: A Description of the Syndrome and Preliminary Findings With Light Therapy. Arch Gen Psychiatry. (1984)

Chapter Two: The Light Effect

In the past century, sunlight has earned a bad reputation for its connection to skin cancer, and several industries have been built around preventing it. As a result many people have stopped asking about sunlight's role in our health and well-being and have started slathering on the sun block. But what if the truth were much different?

THE COLOR FACTOR

Color can have a significant effect on biology, right down to the microscopic level. Humans, animals and plants act and react differently with color changes. John Ott discovered cells change their behavior when colored filters are placed over microscope lights.[37] While these cells acted in specific patterns under natural sunlight conditions, Ott found he could alternate or break up these patterns by using color filters.

It is well established the colors we see are, in fact, varying wavelengths of reflected light. Reflected light and indirect light have a photobiological impact on our health and well-being. Research indicates that pink rooms are soothing, while blue rooms excite and agitate. Bright light exposure can reduce jet lag, and children with mental disabilities learn most quickly in yellow-colored rooms.[38]

To calm violent children, San Bernardino County Probation Department uses a bubble gum pink cell. "[Before the cell] we used to have to literally sit on them," says clinical psychologist Paul E. Boccumini. The room tends to relax the children, and some fall asleep after ten minutes. Despite skepticism from some psychologists, an estimated 1,500 hospitals and correctional institutes across America have placed at least one passive pink room in their facilities.

Many scientists are now convinced light has a far greater impact on health and behavior than previously thought. The ancient and once discredited field of chromo therapy has reinvented itself as "photobiology." Russia is a leader in photobiology, replacing the fluorescent lights in

---

[37] Ott, J., The Effects of Natural and Artificial Light on Man and Other Living Things, (2000)
[38] Birren, F., Color psychology and color therapy: A Factual Study of the influence of color on human life (1961) Gruson, Lindsey, New York Times, Color has a Powerful Effect on Behavior (October 1982)

schoolrooms with full spectrum lamps containing ultraviolet light. As a result, "Children grow faster than usual, work ability and grades are improved and infections are fewer," says Faber Birren, a respected color consultant.

Wohlfarth reported that after changing the school room walls from orange and white to light blue, and installing grey carpet and full spectrum lighting, children's mean systolic blood pressure dropped nearly seventeen percent from 120 to 100. The children were also better behaved, more attentive and less aggressive. Barbara Meister Vitale has worked with both children and color and concluded that color affects hyperactivity in children. In Vitale's studies, placing certain colors in front of children reduced hyperactivity, increased attention span and improved their speed and accuracy in completing assignments. The color of a child's clothing also affected behavior. Vitale learned that color is specific to the individual; the child's favorite color was the most effective in inducing behavioral changes, while the opposite color was least effective.[39]

Color is now being used successfully to enhance children's reading skills. Psychologist Helen Irlen discovered a way to significantly improve learning and behavior in children and adults by placing transparencies and tinted lenses over reading materials in order to block wavelengths causing sensitivity or an adverse effect.[40] Some colors in specific photon wavelengths may cause electrochemical abnormalities in the photoreceptors of the eyes, thus distorting energy signals to the brain.

Irlen claims that some individuals have visual dyslexia or scotopic sensitivity syndrome, a condition caused by light that distorts what the eyes can see. Those affected by this condition respond abnormally to specific wavelengths of light. For example, they may feel overwhelmed in the presence of certain wavelengths. Irlen's system has been successfully adopted by several school systems around the world. A report from The Massachusetts Department of Education in March of 2004 found marked improvement using the Irlen System. The report focused on 4th grade children who were not achieving at expected levels and found when given the appropriate color overlay, "[The children's] reading comprehension score showed a two year increase in only three months."[41] An Irlen Institute review

---

[39] Vitale, B. M., Unicorns Are Real Vitale. (1982)
[40] Fulton, J. T. Process in biological vision including electrochemistry of the neuron. (2009)
[41] Stone, Rhonda. The Light Barrier: Understanding the Mystery of Irlen Syndrome and Light. (2002)

with reports from the United States and Europe also shows compelling success rates.

The photobiological effect of using light on the brain appears promising. Neuroscientist Dr. John Downing also has conducted innovative research on color and ocular stimulation. In one study, he used pulsed and colored light shining through the retina to the hypothalamus which then converted the light to nerve impulses in the brain. According to Downing, these nerve impulses improve brain function and field of vision. This research shows promise for people with learning disabilities by stimulating creativity, memory, motivation and reducing stress.[42]

VISIBLE LIGHT

We tend to take light for granted because we see it every day and it is easy to underestimate its nearly miraculous power. We fail to recognize that light is quite sophisticated and yet not fully understood. The electromagnetic spectrum (EMS), also known as radiant energy, is a range of electromagnetic energy pulses of which our eyes can perceive only a small portion. This small portion is what we call "visible" light. Most electromagnetic radiation consists of wavelengths which are right outside of our visual range, including x-rays, gamma rays, micro waves and radio waves.

Visible light waves are so tiny they have to be measured in nanometers (nm – one nanometer is a billionth of a meter). Some electromagnetic waves are extremely long, such as AM radio waves which can be up to a few football fields long. The other side of the spectrum is x-rays which are extremely short, at about 30 atoms across.

The colors we see are actually the waves that reflect light once it has bounced off of an object. When white light passes through a prism, it appears as a rainbow, the full spectrum of color visible to the eye. Pure sun rays are actually a composite of many colors of visible light. When visible light energy hits matter, depending on the characteristics of the object, certain wavelengths are absorbed and others are reflected. An object appears black when it absorbs all of the radiant wavelengths, while an object appears white when it reflects them. When an object absorbs only portions of the

---

[42] Breiling, Brian. Light Years Ahead: the illustrated guide to full spectrum and colored light in mindbody healing Celestial Arts. (1996)

visible spectrum, we see various colors. For example, when an object reflects red and green light, we see the color yellow.[43]

SUNLIGHT AND VITAMIN D

Sunlight's forgotten healing potential has been reawakened through scientific discovery and photobiological research. In the beginning of the 20th century, people used the sun to treat a number of ailments. Finsen earned his Nobel Prize for treating tuberculosis with UV light. He also studied the effects of UV light on small pox. While UV aggravated the lesions, red light accelerated healing.

During World War I military surgeons used sunlight to disinfect and heal wounds. In the early 1930s, people were encouraged to sunbathe as a public health measure. The sun in combination with fresh air was used for preventing and curing disease. Sunlight as a disinfectant might sound like a strange idea, but history shows women in rural areas used the sun as a natural disinfectant. Mothers taught their daughters to put pillows and rugs out in the sun to sterilize them. More recently, the common practice of using sunlight to sterilize water was tested: using a strict protocol, sunlight combined with oxygen can effectively decontaminate drinking water containing fecal matter.[44]

Architects began designing sunlit buildings that integrated solar ideals. Hospitals were also built with sunlight in mind; special glass was installed to allow maximum UV radiation. However, after the development of antibiotics, the medicinal and hygienic properties of sunlight were no longer considered important.[45]

In contrast, hospitals that are not well-lit by the sun have an increased bacteria level, and unfortunately this has become prevalent, even in the United States. It's a fact hospital-acquired infections are now considered the eight leading cause of death in the world. It's also a fact that sunlight induces several photobiological responses and is capable of killing bacteria, even through glass. "There is evidence that patients in well sunlit wards

---

[43] What Wavelength Goes with a Color?
www.eosweb.larc.nasa.gov/EDDOCS/Wavelengths_for_Colors.html
[44] Reed, R.H. "Solar inactivation of fecal bacteria in water: the critical role of oxygen." Letters in Applied Microbiology. Volume 24, Issue 4, pages 276–280. (April 1997)
[45] Leinhard, John H. *Engines of Our Ingenuity*: No. 1769 Niels Finsen.
www.uh.edu/engines/epi1769.htm

recover faster than their counterparts in room with little or no natural light." [46]

To prove this point, Dr. Auguste Rollier, the director of a sun-therapy clinic in the Swiss Alps, conducted a study involving UV radiation.[47] Rollier ensured his patients received the highest amount of UV light possible. In his book, *Curing with the Sun*, Rollier documents success in treating the following:

- tuberculosis
- colitis
- anemia
- gout
- cystitis
- arteriosclerosis
- rheumatoid arthritis
- eczema
- acne
- lupus
- asthma
- kidney problems

Rollier found, however, the sun's healing rays did not work when his patients wore sunglasses, suggesting the importance of the photobiological nature of our eyes in absorbing sunlight.

Available literature on sunbathing and sunlight exposure is a mass of contradictions; some studies promote its benefits, while others stress its dangers. Sunlight is essential to our health, although paradoxically, it accelerates aging of the skin, can lead to cataracts and may trigger skin cancer in susceptible individuals. The National Institute of Health discovered that limiting exposure to natural sunlight leads to a loss of muscle tone and strength.

Further research shows daily direct exposure to sunlight plays a critical role in children's eye development.[48] Apparently, daylight sends a signal to the brain which affects eye growth. The result of having insufficient exposure to sunlight appears to make nearsightedness more likely, especially

---

[46] Wenzel, Richard P. and Edmund, Michael B. "The Impact of Hospital-Aquired Bloodstream Infections." www.cdc.gov/ncidod/eid/vol7no2/wenzel.htm

[47] Moritz, A., Heal Yourself with Sunlight. (2003)

[48] http://www.npr.org/2011/06/26/137429517/buried-indoors-ranks-of-nearsighted-grow

in those that are genetically predisposed. Interestingly, the University of Vienna's Institute of Human Biology found that the children born in the spring tended to be taller at adulthood than their counterparts born in autumn. Researchers believe that sunlight exposure during the period three months before birth and three months after is especially important and possibility activates an abundant release of human growth hormone.[49]

A lack of sunlight has also been associated with the development of multiple sclerosis (MS). *Neurology Magazine* recently published a study suggesting a lack of sunlight plus a previous illness with mononucleosis can increase the risk of MS.[50]

Has the health care system overlooked the importance of natural light? Could chronic Illness be a symptom of full spectrum light deprivation? In the summer of 1959, John Ott and Jane C. Wright M.D., the physician in charge of cancer research at Bellevue Medical Center in New York City, asked fifteen cancer patients to spend as much time as possible in natural sunlight without their sunglasses. Wright found that fourteen of the fifteen patients had no further advancement in tumor development; in fact several actually showed improvement. One patient did not understand the instructions and wore optical glasses that blocked UV rays. This patient had no positive effect from the sun exposure.[51]

We need to receive a certain amount of light everyday to maintain proper health. Sunlight activates an important biochemical reaction that improves low energy, depression, skin irritations and other ailments. Without sunlight we become "mal-illuminated," according to ophthalmologist Jacob Liberman.[52] For thousands of years we existed in an agricultural economy where most people worked outdoors and got plenty of sunlight, but in 1986, the Bulletin of Atomic Scientists reported that over eighty percent of the workforce is now indoors.[53]

Light may be similar to vitamins and minerals in that humans appear to require a broad spectrum of wavelengths for physical and mental well-being. As we absorb light, different wavelengths seem to go through specific photobiological responses in our mind-body functioning. MIT Professor

---

[49] Hobday, Richard, Ph.D.., The Healing Sun: Sunlight and Health in the 21st Century, Findhorn Press. 2000
[50] Rettner, Rachael, Lack of Sunlight and Mono Infection Combine to Raise MS Risk. (2011)
[51] Ott, John, Health and Light, Packet Book New York. (1973)
[52] Liberman, J., Light: Medicine of the Future, Bear & Company. (1993)
[53] Bulletin of atomic scientists.(April 1986)

Richard Wurtman, M.D. points out, "Specific wavelengths do have biomedical effects on vitamin D production or bilirubin breakdown..."[54] Similar to food, air and water, it appears that light may ignite cellular metabolism and act as a catalyst for crucial processes that transmit messages between the brain and the immune system.

Several studies have shown vitamin D deficiency is estimated to range from a minimum of about fifty percent to over seventy percent in teens and middle-aged people, and between a forty to sixty-five percent deficiency in infants and toddlers. A major cause of vitamin D deficiency is lack of sun exposure. Vitamin D deficiency is now recognized as a pandemic, according to the American Journal of Clinical Nutrition. Few foods naturally contain vitamin D, and foods fortified with vitamin D are often inadequate to satisfy a person's daily requirement.[55] More recent studies published in the *Journal of the National Cancer Institute* indicate a relationship between a lack of vitamin D and risk of some cancers, especially those involving the digestive track such as colon cancer.[56]

Actually, vitamin D is not a vitamin at all, but a naturally occurring pre-hormone that gets activated when sunlight penetrates the skin.[57] As we know nutrition in the form of vitamins and minerals helps people maintain proper health. Sunlight, however, is also a critical part of our diet. Vitamin D (7-dehydrocholestrol hormone) helps with bone growth and density and is known to affect many other biological and physiological factors that are just beginning to be understood. Sunlight activates a 72-hour photobiological process, beginning with 7-dehydrocholestrol and ending up in the liver as dihydroxuyctimin, otherwise referred to as "solitrol." UV-B sunlight in the range of 290-300nm is needed to synthesize vitamin D in our bodies. Under optimal circumstances, our bodies can synthesize up to 20,000 international units (IU) of vitamin D (cholecalciferol) per hour, depending upon the melanin levels in the skin.

Known as a maverick in his field, Dr. William Campbell Douglass is renowned for his photobiological research on treating patients with light. He argues the best way to fight skin cancer is to spend time in direct sunlight—

---

[54] Marte, L. D., Malillumination vs. posillumination: "malillumination" is to "light" as "malnutrition" is to "food".

[55] American Journal of Clinical Nutrition - Vitamin D deficiency: a worldwide problem with health consequences, Vol. 87, No. 4, 1080S-1086S. (April 2008)

[56] Whitworth, A. Low Vitamin D Levels Associated with Increased Total Cancer Incidence. Journal of the National Cancer Institute. 98 (7), 425. (2006)

[57] Cannell J. J. & Hollis B. W., Use of Vitamin D in clinical practice. (2008)

without sunscreen.[58] He cautions people to use common sense and head indoors before they burn, but notes that exposing skin to the sun without any sunscreen is necessary for optimal health. Sunscreen interferes with light absorption and blocks the UV needed for vitamin D synthesis. People who use sun block may actually inhibit their body's normal hormonal synthesis. The time of day you spend outdoors is important, too. The body responds better to sunlight if it is not trying to cool itself down. Sunbathing in morning, evening or on cool days seems to get the best photobiological response.[59]

The pineal gland acts as the body's "light meter." Sunlight is converted by photoreceptor cells into electrical impulses when it enters the eyes. These impulses not only allow for vision, but also trigger the hypothalamus and pineal glands, sending chemical messengers that regulate important hormonal functions throughout the body. The pineal gland controls the sympathetic and parasympathetic nervous systems that regulate hormonal balance and control secretions of the pituitary gland and endocrine system. The hypothalamus coordinates and regulates many of our life-sustaining functions. These secretions govern most bodily functions, including the immune system, digestion, sexual function and moods.[60]

Ultraviolet radiation in sunlight activates the release of vitamin D and is then stored in the body for several weeks. Studies found that vitamin D works as a protective agent against autoimmune diseases and some forms of cancer.[61] Vitamin D helps regulate the balance of calcium and phosphorous necessary for bone formation and remodeling. It also increases the body's ability to absorb magnesium. When vitamin D levels are low, the body cannot absorb enough calcium to stay healthy, regardless of the amount ingested. Calcium is essential for DNA synthesis, a healthy immune system, teeth and bone growth.

According to the *Washington Post*, vitamin D deficiency is becoming more prevalent, in some cases leading to rickets in children and possibly osteoporosis in the elderly. This research has sparked a heated debate

---

[58] Douglass, William, Campbell, Into the Light: Tomorrow's Medicine Today! (2003)
[59] Garland, Cedric F., French, Christine B., Baggerly, Leo L, and Heaney, Robert P. "Vitamin D Supplement Doses and Serum 25-Hydroxyvitamin D in the Range Associated with Cancer Prevention" Anti-Cancer Research 31: 607-612. (2011)
[60] Liberman, J. LIGHT: Medicine of the Future. (1991)
[61] Norris, M. J. Can the Sunshine Vitamin Shed Light on Type 1 Diabetes? (2001)

between advocates and critics of spending more time outdoors.[62] In cases of vitamin D deficiency, a mother's breast milk does not contain enough vitamin D to meet an infant's needs. Recently, there has been a rise in rickets among children that has caused health officials to become concerned. Moreover, a deficiency of vitamin D can cause osteomalacia, a softening of the bones in adults. *Contra Costa Times* staff writer Suzanne Bohan interviewed several scientists and doctors from around the country and discovered that leading nutritionists at Children's Hospital in Oakland, California believe there is a widespread vitamin D deficiency in the United States, leading to poor immune systems and brain function, among other conditions.[63]

It is possible that vitamin D plays an underappreciated role in preventing nearly every major disease afflicting Western societies. Vitamin D has been found to assist in the prevention of the following:

- high blood pressure
- heart attack
- congestive heart failure
- stroke
- type 2 diabetes
- muscle weakness
- osteoporosis

Vitamin D also supports mood stability, especially in older people, and may play a role in the prevention and/or treatment of the following health conditions:

- asthma
- atherosclerosis
- bladder cancer
- breast cancer
- chronic fatigue syndrome
- colon cancer
- Crohn's disease

---

[62] Rajakumar, MD, Kumaravel. Vitamin D, Cod-Liver Oil, Sunlight, and Rickets: A Historical Perspective. Pediatrics. 112(2), 132-135. (2003)
[63] Bohan, Suzzanne. Vitiman D Sees The Light 'Sunshine' nutrient may have key role in halting disease. Contra Costa Times. (2008)

- ovarian cancer
- depression
- epilepsy
- fibromyalgia
- heart attack
- hypertension
- inflammatory bowel disease
- kidney disease
- liver disease
- multiple sclerosis
- periodontal disease
- preeclampsia
- psoriasis
- rectal cancer
- rheumatoid arthritis
- senile dementia

Vitamin D also assists in the lowering the risk of inflammation and bacterial infections.[64] Researchers have found exposure to sunlight is similar to exercise in its effect on the body, improving blood pressure and increasing oxygen in our cells. Dr. Zane Kime's book, *Sunlight,* states that continual exposure to sunlight produces beneficial photobiological responses, including an increase in heart rate, respiratory rate and lactic acid in the blood flow similar to those produced by physical exercise.[65] Kime also found increases in energy, muscle strength, endurance, vitality, mental stability and a higher tolerance for stress. He noted that blood absorbs more oxygen when exposed to sunlight and concluded, "The most biologically active part of sunlight is UV rays, which are absolutely critical for optimal health." For example, most individuals who live at high altitudes or in equatorial regions exhibit lower rates of cancer and it is believed to be due to the abundance of UV rays.

Ultraviolet radiation also plays an integral role in the body's cholesterol breakdown process. Sunlight exposure can have a significant photobiological effect on cholesterol levels, and seasonal changes have been associated with blood pressure. Nearly 100 million people suffer from high

---

[64] www.whfoods.org/genpage.php?tname=nutrient&dbid=110vitamin D
[65] Kime, Z. Sunlight. City: World Health Pubns. (1980)

blood pressure, costing healthcare systems billions of dollars each year. There is a clear correlation between the rise of cholesterol and blood pressure levels, the farther one lives from the equator. This rise becomes more significant during the winter when solar radiation is at its lowest.[66]

Furthermore, people with darker complexions living far from the equator experience higher incidences of hypertension than those with lighter complexions.[67] African American adults are estimated to be two to three times more likely to have a vitamin D deficiency than Caucasian adults. Put simply, individuals with dark complexions (higher levels of melanin) require more sunlight to photosynthesize vitamin D than fair-skinned people.

By far the most important contributing factor to vitamin D deficiency all over the world is insufficient exposure to sunlight. The exact amount of vitamin D required for optimum health has not been accurately determined, nor has the amount of sun exposure necessary to reach a sufficient level. In recent years, the Recommended Daily Allowance (RDA) for vitamin D has been raised. The current public health recommendations for vitamin D published by the Institute of Medicine at the National Academy of Sciences recommend 400 to 800 IU per day. In cases where vitamin D is used as a treatment or therapy, as much as 10,000 to 50,000 IU per day may be administered. The National Academy of Sciences has also set tolerable upper intake levels for vitamin D as follows: [68]

- Infants, 0-6 months: 1,000 IU per day
- 6-12 months: 1,500 IU per day
- 1-3 years: 2,500 IU per day
- 4-8 year: 3,000 IU per day
- 9-18 years: 4,000 IU per day
- Adults, 19 years and older: 4,000 IU per day
- Pregnant and lactating women: 4,000 IU per day

There is a synthetic versus natural supplement debate regarding vitamin D supplements. Vitamin D can also be obtained from food, animal or microbial sources. Natural vitamin D3 supplements are commonly

---

[66] Colpo, A., LDL Cholesterol: Bad' Cholesterol, or Bad Science? (2005)

[67] Rostand, S.G., Ultraviolet Light May Contribute to Geographic and Racial Blood Pressure Differences. (1997)

[68] www.iom.edu/Reports/2010/Dietary-Reference-Intakes-for-Calcium-and-Vitamin-D/Report-Brief.aspx

produced from lanolin and/or fish products. Food sources of vitamin D include the following: [69]

• salmon	(100 grams)	411 IU
• prawns/shrimp	(100 grams)	160 IU
• sardines	(1 can - 80 grams)	250 IU
• cod	(100 grams)	63 IU
• eggs	(per one egg)	23 IU

Preventative and interactive medicine begins with skeptical inquiry into what impacts our health. If we want to build a healthier society, we have to research and ask questions. We cannot rely on doctors to stay current with all areas of research; we must be proactive.

HUMAN BIOPHOTONS

It has been proven that all living cells emit light. The small fraction of light a living cell emanates has been termed "biophoton." This term comes from the Greek, with bio meaning "life" and photon meaning "light" (not to be confused with "bioluminescence," the energy released by fireflies, angelfish and other creatures). Biophotonics is the science of interactions and emanations of light within living cells. This phenomenon has various scientific names:

- biophoton
- biofields
- bioelectromagnetics
- low level biological chemiluminescence
- ultra weak photon emissions (UPE)
- mitogenetic radiation/rays
- bioelectromagnetics
- dark luminescence
- photobiological energy

---

[69] www.naturopath.co.nz/Articles/Nutritional+Medicine/Vitamins+And+Minerals/Vitamins/Vitamin+D.html

Biophotonic energy might be the driving force for all the molecules in the human body. The cell emanates the most light during cell birth and death. Any change in the biological or physiological state of the living system is reflected in the biophoton emission. Scientific studies conclude injured cells will emit a higher biophotonic signal than normal cells, and any disturbance in the biological system increases the production of photons. When a cell is distressed, its biophotonic signal shines brighter, as if it is screaming out to other cells for help.

Biophotonics is a rapidly increasing field of current scientific research. Today scientists affiliated with the International Institute of Biophysics in Neuss, Germany, are continuing to discover new data on biophotons. The research includes non-invasive methods of investigating biological tissues. The Institute's goal is to apply the understanding of biophotonics within a theoretical framework to medicine, pharmacology, science and the food industry.[70]

Scientists have been researching biophotonics for nearly a century. While developing a method for cancer diagnosis in 1923, Russian scientist Alexander Gurwitsch encountered ultra-weak photon emissions from living tissues and introduced the concept of a morphogenetic field.[71] Gurwitsch called these emissions "mitogenetic radiation" and was convinced the rays of light were connected to cell division. He was criticized for his discovery because other scientists had difficulty replicating the findings.

Other evidence supporting Gurwitsch's hypothesis rests with Kirlian photography, developed in 1940 by Russian inventor and electrician, Seymon Kirlian, making it possible to view the kinetic energy fields surrounding living organisms.[72] Here, subjects are photographed in electrical fields of high frequency, high voltage and low amperage, producing an image that appears as a number of small sparks or miniature lightning-type patterns outlining the subject. (A famous example of a Kirlian technique photograph is the image of a hand outlined with light during the opening credits of *The X-Files*). While little photobiological research has been done to follow up on Kirlian's work, advocates believe these photographs can document emotional and physical changes determined by colors and patterns.

---

[70] Bischof, M. Biophotonen. Zweitauseneins. (1996)
[71] The History of Bioresonance Therapy - www.stmaryclinic.com/all_about_bio.htm
[72] Schmeidler, G. & Kirlian photography history. (2007)

Currently Kirlian photography is being researched as a medical diagnostic tool.[73] In 1964 Russian scientist Yu A. Valdimirov found wavelengths of super-weak metabolic luminance range from ultraviolet 360nm to infrared 800nm.[74] He believed these light emanations could be used for medical diagnosis. Scientists and physicians working in the General Hospital in Madras, India, also recognize this application.[75] They believe the fields act as fingerprints that can identify certain physical disorders and conditions, including brain tumors. Could the ability to detect human bio-magnetic fields become the most accurate diagnostic tool in medicine?

Founding Director of the Center for Frontier Science Beverly Rubik, Ph.D. believes we are naturally equipped with antennae and radiators for biofields, and her research has uncovered some interesting constructs about this phenomenon. [76] She states, "Biofields are fields surrounding living biological objects." A fifty-two week study conducted in South Korea found the subjects' bio-emission rates were at their lowest in autumn. The experiments also found that all people have a chronobiological order, or consistent rhythmic light patterns. Another study found that after meditation, the human biophotonic signature was at its lowest (calmest), providing the lowest photon count. This study also indicated that meditation reduces free-radical reaction and has a positive effect on people's health.

It is thought that free-radical reactions are partially responsible for higher biophotonic (light) emissions. This light is measured in photons per square centimeter per second. It has been found the abdomen, lower back and chest emit approximately 4 photons per second (PPS), a person's forehead 23 PPS, while the hands emit about 27 PPS. These measurements were made by Dr. Jessel-Kenyon in the U.K., using a photomultiplier. He also found symmetry in the photon readings from both sides of the body in healthy people, but unhealthy people showed distinct asymmetry in their readings.

In *The Field*, Lynne McTaggart hypothesizes that each cellular emission is like a musical instrument, imperceptible as a single unit and

[73] Stanwick, M. "Aura Photography: Mundane Physics or Diagnostic Tool?" Nursing Times. (1996)

[74] Yu. A. Valdimirov, Bessonova, T. S., Stanislavskii, M. P., Khaimov-Mal' , V. Ya. and G. V. Molev, Spectra and radioluminescence kinetics of doped corundum crystals. (1964)

[75] Therapeutic magnetism yesterday and today, magnetic healing through the ages. www.quantumbalancing.com/news/magnetic.htm

[76] Rubik, B., The Biofield Hypothesis: Its Biophysical Basis and Role in Medicine. (2002)

creating a harmonic symphony of light or "multitude of tuning forks that all begin resonating together."

In separate biophotonic research, University of Arizona Professors Katherine Creath and Melinda H. Connor each made interesting observations. Creath found "halo-like" energy captured in images of plant leaves. "Biophotonic chemiluminescence emission persists as a by-product of metabolic function." As the leaves dry up, the biophotonic emission continues and even slightly increases. Connor made a connection between the biophoton and healing, using human subjects, focusing on "healing intention" of living organic matter.[77]

Biophoton theory suggests that light is stored in DNA, more precisely at the cells' nuclei. This was observed when the ultra-weak photoemission stopped appearing after removal of the cell nuclei.[78] Biophotic researchers believe a communication network acts via an electromagnetic field of interactions, creating a messaging system between an organism and its environment.

It was first hypothesized that biophotic actions were part of the cellular communication process by German theoretical biophysicist Fritz-Albert Popp in 1970. Popp coined the term "biophoton" and was the first to address the idea of light's coherence.

In the quantum world, "coherence" means subatomic particles that exist in a coordinated state— a condition of subatomic waves or particles being in the same phase or going the same direction. Marco Bischof has gotten attention because of his 2005 book, *Biophotons: The Light in Our Cells*. According to Bischof, "This radiation is very weak, but it is not like an ordinary light, because it is coherent. Like laser light, but is much more coherent than any laser that is possible to make." [79]

He and his team produced considerable evidence proving biophotonic emission is associated with photobiological and physiological function when they found molecules in cells responded to certain light wavelength. By 1974, Dr. V.P. Kazmacheyev in Novosibirsk, Russia had

---

[77] Maret, K., Energy Medicine in the United States: Historical Roots and the Current Status. (2009)

[78] Da Nóbrega, C. A. M., Biophoton – The language of the cells what can living systems tell us about interaction? (2003)

[79] Bishop, M., Biophotons -The Light in Our Cells. (2005)

detected intercellular communication by means of these mytogenic rays, thus confirming Popp's theories.[80]

In one instance, Popp's work was verified by one of his critics. Bernard Ruth was an experimental physicist who thought Popp's ideas were ridiculous and wanted to debunk his hypothesis.[81] Ruth asked Popp to serve as his advisor in designing a machine that revealed cellular light, believing he would fail. Popp ultimately developed a photomultiplier that accurately counted photons, thus verifying his hypothesis. For decades that photomultiplier remained the most effective tools in measuring cellular photon emissions on the planet.

In 2009 researchers elaborated on Popp's studies, indicating light may be used as a way for cells to communicate as photonic electromagnetic waves that influence each other at a distance, and then become drawn to each other if vibrating out of phase. Popp called this exchange of photons between living entities "photon sucking,"[82] and realized this exchange might answer some of the animal kingdom's most persistent conundrums: how schools of fish or flocks of birds create perfect and instantaneous coordination, for example. Many experiments on the homing ability of animals demonstrate it has nothing to do with following habitual trails, scents, or even the electromagnetic fields of the earth, but rather some form of silent communication that acts like an invisible rubber band, binding these animals together, even when they are separated by great distance.

Experiments in cellular communication were performed wherein two groups of cells were selected from the same culture. One cell culture was used as the initiation sample and was subjected to a chemical poison. The second cell culture was left unaltered in order to observe any transmitted effects from the culture sample being killed. A window was placed between the two samples. There were several thousand photobiological experiments conducted, all in total darkness. When the window between the two cell samples was made of ordinary glass, the second sample remained alive and healthy. When the window was made of quartz, the second sample became ill and died with the same symptoms as the poisoned sample, even though it

---

[80] V.P. Kaznacheyev, L.P. Mikhailova, Sverkhslabye, Izlucheniya, V., Mezhkletochnykh, Vzaimodeistviyakh, Nauka. (1981)

[81] Valone, T. F., Bioelectromagnetic Healing, its History and a Rationale for its Use. (2003)

[82] Bajpai, R.P., Popp, F.A., van Wijk, R., Niggli, H., Beloussov, L.V., Cohen, S., Jung, H.H., Sup-Soh, K., Lipkind, M., Voiekov, V.L., Slawinski, J., Aoshima, Y., Michiniewicz, Z., van Klitzing, L., Swain, J.:Biophotons Indian Journal of Experimental Biology 41, Vol 5, 391-544. (2003)

had not been exposed to the toxin. The major transmission difference between glass and quartz is that quartz transmits both UV and infrared well, while ordinary glass does not.[83]

Professors Herbert A. Pohl and Joe S. Crane did extensive work on the emissions of weak radio signals from the cells of humans, animals, plants and bacteria. They found radio signals were always highest during cell division. [84] Based on these findings, the emissions had a purpose to communicate within the body, but potentially, between living things as well.

Is it possible that biological radiation is part of a deeper collective order in regulating organisms? It does sound a bit like science fiction to think of cells communicating with micro lasers. It will be interesting to see how future of biophotonic science and technology unfolds. This new understanding could have a major impact on how science views photobiology, how the medical industry treats illness and how diagnoses are made, in addition to finding new ways of responding to and eradicating disease.

ARTIFICIAL LIGHT

Artificial light sources can be toxic to our bodies. Light combinations or the lack of certain wavelengths can be harmful, compromising the immune system. Standard fluorescent bulbs cause iron in the blood to coagulate, which can contribute to blood clots. Decades of research continually point to the negative photobiological effects produced by artificial lighting.[85]

Incandescent light bulbs emit a limited range of visible colors; they are commonly deficient on the blue end of the spectrum and emit virtually no UV light. Florescent bulbs, however, can produce a different range of light depending on the phosphors (florescent gases) in the tubes. Placing specific phosphors can actually yield the closest to a solar match.[86] For an additional cost, florescent tubes can be enhanced to wide spectrum, or upgrade further what's known as full spectrum, which is the closest solar match. LED full spectrums are undeniably the best form of artificial light.

---

[83] Trushin, M.V., The possible role of electromagnetic fields in bacterial communication. (2003)
[84] Pohl, H. A. & Crane, J. S. , Dielectrophoresis of cells. (1971)
[85] Veitch, J. A. & McColl S. L., Full spectrum Fluorescent Lighting Effects on People: A Critical Review. (2001)
[86] The science of light http://www.scribd.com/doc/37809265/Learn-Lightening

Dr. Fritz Hollwich in 1980 conducted a study of people working under cool white florescent light and found high levels of the stress hormones ACTH and cortisol.[87] These hormones function as growth inhibitors and possibly stunt growth in children. Hollwich saw these stress hormones were absent in individuals under sunlight-simulated florescent tubes, which confirmed the biological importance of full spectrum lighting. In addition to those factors is fluorescent tube flicker (a consequence of its 60 hertz per second cycle). All of the issues have been linked to:

- headaches
- eye-strain
- fatigue
- epileptic seizures

With the recent adaptation of the electronic ballast, the flicker rate can be easily resolved, and electronic ballast has become the industry standard in new construction. In response to the harmful effects of fluorescent lighting, the Germans adopted this technology, outfitting their hospitals with full spectrum lights.

Suffering from his own ailments of arthritis and a degenerative hip problem, Ott applied his ideas to himself. He began his personal photobiological treatment by avoiding sunglasses and spending as much time in the sun as he could. His "light" diet resulted in less painful arthritis and hip improvement; x-rays backed up his claims of improved health. A friend of Ott's who had blood vessels burst in his eyes went nearly blind, but six months after Ott suggested that he expose himself to more sunlight, he was able to see color again and could trace the vague outline of a sidewalk.

A U.S. Navy melanoma study discovered personnel who worked indoors had a higher risk of melanoma than their counterparts working outside, an unexpected finding.[88] The study also revealed melanoma occurred on the trunk of the body more often than the head or arms, the latter two of which are commonly exposed to sunlight. Other research shows breast cancer is five times more common in industrialized than in unindustrialized

---

[87] Martel, L. D., Scientific discoveries about the human eye suggest blue light to improve health, learning, and workplace performance. (2005)

[88] Martin R., White, MPH, Frank C. Garland Ph D. Malignant Melanoma in US Navy Personnel Naval Health Research Center, San Diego, California. (1989)

nations, a fact that leads to the belief artificial lighting might contribute to this epidemic.

Our bodies depend upon the rhythms of light and dark. A lack of sunlight may affect physiological and psychological functions, including fertility and mood.[89] The circadian rhythm is more than an inner clock; circadian disruption may alter hormonal secretions. Studies have shown women who work the night shift have a nearly fifty percent higher risk for breast cancer than those who work during the day.[90] At Thomas Jefferson Medical School in Philadelphia, Dr. George Brainard found in an environment of artificial light, abnormal secretions of various hormones such as:

- melatonin
- testosterone
- cortisone
- lymphocyte cells
- thyroid hormones

Scientists have concluded that office workers are twice as likely to develop skin cancer, while those who work outdoors have the lowest risk. An article from the British medical journal, *Lancet*, in August 1982 reports a study on the photobiological relationship between melanoma and the sun's UV rays that found instances of malignant melanomas were considerably higher in indoor employees than in individuals regularly exposed to sunlight. Dr. Helen Shaw, an assistant researcher with the project, discovered the individuals with the lowest risk of developing melanoma were those who spent time sunbathing. In addition, office employees who worked under traditional artificial lighting had twice the risk of developing melanomas. Shaw also noted that animal cells exposed to standard florescent light developed mutations. A later study confirmed the correlation between melanoma and fluorescent lights.[91]

In addition, full spectrum lighting increases productivity and concentration. For example, children's classroom attention improves under

---

[89] Vitaterna, M. H., Takahashi, J. S., and Turek, F. W., Overview of Circadian Rhythms.
[90] West, Larry. Light Pollution Raises Risk of Breast Cancer
[91] Jensen, A. A. Melanoma, Fluorescent Lights, and Polychlorinated Biphenyls. The Lancet, 320, 935. (1982)

full spectrum lighting.[92] The larger range of light wavelengths can nullify the effects of hyperactivity.[93] Obrig Laboratories, a Florida company of about 100 employees, installed full spectrum lighting in the 1970's.   Work production increased by nearly twenty-five percent. In addition, a flu epidemic in the area did not impact any of its employees.[94]

Artificial light also affects also dental health. A finding by the Sarasota County Dental Society show children in classrooms under radiation-shielded full spectrum florescent lights developed one-third the number of cavities as their classmates in classrooms without these special lights.[95] Researchers at the University of Chicago Dental Clinic conducted experiments showing a clear relationship between light and tooth decay in lab animals, which increased or decreased depending upon each creature's light environment.[96]

Research conducted in the 1930's on a large number of children showed the occurrence of cavities was much higher during the school year than during the summer.[97] Furthermore, the number of cavities was directly related to the amount of sunlight where the children lived; more sunlight equated to fewer cavities. What exact role did sunlight play in these results?

These are just a few of the ways light has been shown to impact our health and well-being. As participants in the health care system, we owe it to ourselves and our children to understand how our health relates to our environment. Sunlight, like food and water, is a fundamental element of good health. In our societal search for solutions and answers, we may have temporarily lost this simple idea. Fortunately, through visionaries, research, discussion and exploration, we can widen this avenue of preventative medicine and enrich our ability to recover, maintain and nourish our own bodies.

---

[92] Marte, L. D., Malillumination vs. Posillumination: "Malillumination" is to "light" as "malnutrition" is to "food".
[93] Ott. J. N., School Lighting and Hyperactivity. (1980)
[94] Ott, J. The Effects of Natural and Artificial Light on Man and Other Living Things. (2000)
[95] Ott, J., The light side of health. (1986)
[96] Ott, J., Light and health. (1973)
[97] Hathaway, W. E., A Study Into the Effects of Types of Light on Children - A Case of Daylight Robbery. (1992)

Chapter Three: Therapeutic Light Treatments

The photobiological treatments presented here, many of which are FDA-approved, have been researched by credible professionals and academics within the scientific community. We have come to a crossroads in medicine, and now we need to move towards the light. The following is a short list of technology that can rapidly advance healthcare:

- Full Spectrum Light
- LED and Laser Biostimulation
- Photodynamic Therapy
- Blood Irradiation
- Optical Brain Stimulation

FULL SPECTRUM LIGHT

Full spectrum is a therapy to replace the sun for people who live where sunlight is lacking, and for those who work in an office or at night. This therapy can also be used for those who just don't get outside enough. Light ignites neurotransmitters that regulate hormonal function and maintain health.

Ott suggested humans need between thirty minutes and two hours of unobstructed ambient sunlight per day in order to maintain optimum health. Sunglasses and tinted windows prevent full absorption. Eyeglasses and contact lenses block certain wavelengths. Ott's research indicates that sunglasses and sunscreen also block UV light and may severely weaken the body's defenses if used regularly. He once noted, "A car requires fuel, oxygen and a spark to create internal combustion which makes the car run. The human body also requires fuel in the form of food, oxygen and a spark in the form of light to ignite the process of metabolism."

Ott believed light should be treated in the same manner as diet and exercise, and it is important to receive an RDA of light. Low levels of light are not enough to synthesize vitamin D. Using "sunlight" florescent tubes that generate at least 10,000 lux (lux is the measure unit of illumination perceived by the human eye) at a light temperature of 5500k to 6500k (Kelvin scale of light and thermodynamic temperature measurement) from fifteen minutes to an hour per day can be an effective treatment for the symptoms of malillumination. It is best used in the morning to stop production melatonin and trigger serotonin production.

Individuals with high blood pressure were part of a UVB exposure study. The participant's UVB exposure increased when using tanning beds for 30 minutes at three times a week. The study showed a significant increase raised their vitamin D levels by 180 percent and lowered their blood pressure by about five percent.[98]

The sun's natural rays deliver 40,000 to 100,000 lux at 5,600k to 6,500k. In comparison, artificial light in commercial buildings with uncovered windows only reached 300 to 500 lux, whereas a common living room reaches 50 to 200 lux. Light levels on night-shift jobs can be even lower. An overcast or rainy day will emit between 900 to 1200 lux, which can definitely lead to symptoms of SAD and possibly the following:

- general depression
- premenstrual syndrome
- bulimia
- anorexia
- drug addiction
- alcohol addiction

In these cases individuals have experienced a reduction or elimination of their symptoms when exposed to bright, full spectrum light.

NASA has begun to use full spectrum light treatments on astronauts to help them adjust their biological rhythms in space. In addition, travelers have found success treating jet lag with full spectrum light exposure. Dr. Barbara Parry of San Diego, California, has shown that woman respond well to two-hour sessions of bright light treatment in alleviating premenstrual syndrome (PMS) symptoms. Full spectrum lighting is also useful in commercial and home settings, as it presents less eyestrain than incandescent and standard florescent light.[99]

---

[98] http://www.whfoods.com/genpage.php?tname=nutrient&dbid=110
[99] Parry, B.L., Berga, S.L., Kripke, D.F., et. al. Altered Waveform of Plasma Nocturnal Melatonin Secretion in Premenstrual Depression. (1990)

Ott conducted full spectrum lighting studies on the effects of lighting on school age children. The installation of special radiation-shielded, full spectrum lights in schools resulted in:

- significant reduction in behavioral problems
- learning disability reduction
- improved academic performance

The results of Ott's study found several extremely hyperactive children with confirmed learning disabilities calmed down and rapidly overcame their learning and reading problems when exposed to full spectrum lighting. Evidence showed that under the full spectrum light, kids tested higher, grew faster and had two-thirds less cavities.

A Pacific Gas and Electric study said elementary students under natural lighting conditions performed twenty-six percent higher in reading and twenty percent higher in math.[100] Test results were analyzed from three school districts: Capistrano in California, Fort Collins in Colorado and in Seattle, Washington. Other studies include:

- *Brain/Mind Bulletin*, September 1993 "Full spectrum Light Outshines in Classrooms"
- *The Lancet*, November 1987 "Full spectrum Classroom and Sickness in Pupils"
- *Sacramento Bee*, June 1999 "Sunlight Could Perk up Kids' Grades"
- *Washington Post*, November 1999 "Study Says Natural Classroom Lighting Can Aid Achievement".

In this modern world we all spend most of our lives indoors, there is no denying it. Could serious illness be connected to something as simple as that? It's clear that natural light is important to health, and possible much more significant than any of us could of imagined. Life evolves under sunlight, so it makes sense that the sun would play a significant role in our health.

---

[100] Heschong Mahone Group, Daylighting in Schools. (1999)

POWER OF ULTRAVIOLET

For eons nature has used the sun's ultraviolet (UV) energy as a way to cleanse the earth. UV light has many practical uses. As mentioned, UV light is an important factor in health and has also found a niche in many business applications. The following is a list of the many wavelengths of UV light:

- UVA   Ultraviolet A, long wave (black light)   400–315nm
- NUV   Near   400–300nm
- UVB   Ultraviolet B or medium wave   315–280nm
- MUV   Middle   300–200nm
- UVC   Ultraviolet C, short wave, or germicidal   280–100nm
- FUV   Far   200–122nm
- EUV   Extreme   200– 10nm

Ultraviolet light has properties that keep medical instruments sterile, thus playing an integral role in medical facilities worldwide. Maternity wards use what is called "blue light therapy" for the treatment of hyperbilirubinemia (bilirubin), or neonatal jaundice. This condition is found in over sixty percent of prematurely born infants and if left untreated can cause brain damage or even death. Luckily, jaundice-causing bilirubin is easily eliminated from the body with exposure to UV light, full spectrum light or sunlight. The treatment for jaundice was discovered in 1956, and blue light is now used in hospitals around the world for affected babies.[101]

Ott had concerns about UV overexposure when he dined in a Chicago restaurant lit with ultraviolet black-lights. He wondered if the light might have a negative impact on the employees. After asking the restaurant manager a few questions, he learned the employees' health and attendance record had been so good that the hotel management had conducted a formal inquiry to understand why even during flu epidemics, the restaurant employees never got sick. Could there be a photobiological connection between exposure to black lights and good health?

Effects are observed in the animal kingdom as well. When standard florescent lights are replaced with full spectrum lights, zoo animals become more active. Studies have also shown that animals not producing offspring in

---

[101] Cremer, R.J., Perryman, P.W., and Richards, D.H. Influence of light on the hyperbilirubinaemia of infants. (1958)

captivity began to mate when a full spectrum lighting system containing UV was installed.[102] When black lights were placed over some of the fish tanks at the Miami Seaquarium, the curator noticed a decrease in the fatal disease called "pop-eye" (exophthalmus) prevalent in some fish. The curator later reported that certain fish unable to adapt to captivity now thrived under this added ultraviolet light. Similar reports have been published regarding reptiles, birds and animals in zoos throughout the world.[103]

Ultraviolet light is also used in water purification, sewage treatment and air ventilation systems in hospitals and office buildings. The following is a list of UV light applications and their wavelengths:

- 230–400nm: optical sensors
- 230–365nm: label tracking, identification
- 240–280nm: water purification, disinfecting/decontamination (UVGI)
- 250–300nm: forensic analysis, drug detection
- 254nm: air purification, ultraviolet blood irradiation
- 270–300nm: protein analysis, DNA sequencing, drug discovery
- 280–400nm: medical imaging of cells
- 300–400nm: offset printing plates, solid-state lighting
- 300–365nm: curing of polymers
- 315–400nm: psoriasis treatment
- 320–400nm: blood cleaning for transfusions (Cerus Corporation)
- 350–370nm: insect zappers
- 365–400nm: counterfeit money detection
- 405nm: blue ray DVD players
- 420–448nm: neonatal jaundice treatment
- 450–490nm: dental curing light

Recent studies show worker illness and respiratory problems decreased after installing full spectrum lighting in commercial and industrial work environments.[104] In her article "UV Lamps Could Reduce Worker Sickness," Emma Ross points out how new research proves ultraviolet germicidal irradiation (UVGI) removes airborne pathogens in ventilation systems, killing germs and thereby reducing illness.[105]

---

[102]Laszlo, J. Observations on two new artificial lights for reptile displays. International Zoo Yearbook, 9 , 12-13. (1969).

[103] Ott, J. Health And Light. (1973)

[104] Lind, S., Mimicking Daylight with Artificial Light: Upgrading Lighting to Improve Productivity, Safety and Sales in the Workplace. (2010)

[105] Ross, E. UV Lamps Could Reduce Worker Sickness. (2003)

The *Lancet* published an article in which Canadian scientists found a forty percent drop in breathing problems where the UVGI technique was used. It also reduced overall worker sickness by about twenty percent. "The cost of UVGI installation could in the long run prove cost-effective compared with the yearly losses from absence because of building-related illness," says Dr. Dick Menzies, Director of the Respiratory Division at McGill University in Montreal, Canada. He feels the installation of UVGI in North American office buildings could resolve millions of work-related employee illnesses.[106]

Wladyslaw Jan Kowalski, an architectural engineer at Pennsylvania State University's Indoor Environment Center, feels Menzies' study could be a landmark in proving the technique is cost-effective in combatting contagious diseases, such as influenza, in commercial office buildings. "Theoretically, if a large number of schools, office buildings and residences were modified, a number of airborne respiratory diseases could be eradicated by interrupting the transmission cycle," reports Kowalski in his book, *Aerobiological Engineering Handbook A Guide to Airborne Disease Control Technologies.* He asserts, "Reducing the transmission rate sufficiently would... halt epidemics in their path." Poor indoor air quality negatively affects the health of millions in the United States— the potential benefit is huge. If used in school buildings, this technology could have an even larger impact on children. Because they breathe faster than adults, children inhale fifty percent more air per pound of body weight than adults and are especially sensitive to air quality problems.[107]

Companies marketing UVGI technology make some astounding claims about the effectiveness of their technology. Guardian Air has U.S. Environmental Protection Agency (EPA) approved systems. Their independent lab tests indicate their systems kill ninety-nine percent of airborne and surface bacteria, viruses and mold, and eighty-five percent of gases odors, and volatile organic compounds.

---

[106] Menzies, D., Popa, J., Hanley, J.A., Rand, T., & Milton, D.K. Effect of ultraviolet germicidal lights installed in office ventilation systems on workers' health. (2003)
[107] Kowalski, W.J., Aerobiological Engineering Handbook: A Guide to Airborne Disease Control Technologies. (2006)

Their photobiological systems are used in:

- government buildings
- schools
- hospitals
- nursing homes
- cruise ship restaurant chains
- daycare centers
- commercial buildings
- homes

UV light medical applications are also gaining widespread attention. Psoriasis, a skin disorder, can be treated by using UVA in combination with PUVA, a light sensitive compound. One that has been developed is 8-Methoxypsoralen (MOP-8) and was introduced 1978 to be applied topically in conjunction with UV treatment. MOP-8 is a chemical found naturally in figs as a defense against insects; when an insect eats the fruit, it becomes light sensitive and gets burned by the sun.

The use of psoralen is currently part of an FDA-approved system that cleans blood of bacteria and viruses. Cerus Corporation has developed amotosalen, a light-activated psoralen compound which is used to neutralize pathogens in blood for transfusions. The blood is cleaned by mixing it with amotosalen, then exposing it to UV light. John Hearst, Founding Director of Cerus Corporation, Professor Emeritus UC Berkeley, formerly a Senior Staff Scientist at the Lawrence Berkeley National Laboratory and past President of American Society for Photobiology notes that unlike testing procedures, this blood safety method does not rely upon identification of harmful organisms, but cleans the blood of all pathogens during the process, thus guaranteeing safety.[108]

The applications of UV light in maintaining healthy environments, water systems, hospital operation rooms, our skin, our babies and the air we breathe make UV a great tool, and I'm sure many of its uses have yet to be seen.

---

[108] Hurst, J, Interview - Concord, California. (2003)

LED AND LASER BIOSTIMULATION

Biostimulation uses light to accelerate the healing of injured tissue, decrease inflammation and swelling, reduce pain and increase circulation by quickly bringing cells back to their natural state. Currently, biostimulation is the only known successful treatment for diabetic lesions, and in some cases, can save peoples' limbs.

Biostimulation light treatment is effective for:
- wound healing acceleration
- sports injuries
- sciatica
- heals diabetic lesions
- pain management
- helps heal torn ligaments
- eases chronic pain
- supports tissue regeneration
- tendons
- arthritis
- bone fractures
- cartilage damage
- carpal tunnel syndrome
- inflammation and swelling resolution
- bone regeneration in periodontal pockets
- ligament tears
- nerve damage
- oral ulcers
- non-healing wounds
- non-healing fractures

Photobiological studies using biostimulation indicate only one occasional side effect: an increase in discomfort for a short period after treating chronic conditions. However as the body regains balance, the issue resolves itself.

Treatments can last from a few minutes to almost an hour per session. The energy is absorbed by the cell, which causes increased circulation and oxygen flow while removing toxins. Light therapy emits an energy that helps the body with natural healing, enhancing healthy cells and stimulating damaged and irregular cell tissue into an accelerated healing process. Biostimulation works on the affected area (abnormal cell tissue) by irradiating it with a small range of light waves. The light is then absorbed by the photoreceptors within each cell. Photons strike the damaged tissue, creating a cellular response that triggers a physiological response and jump-starts the healing process.

"Light photons are absorbed into cell tissue. Inside of cell tissue there are little molecules called photoreceptor molecules and these are like little radio receivers. It has been found fewer wavelengths shining together coherently activate a better response on tissue," said David Olszewski, electrical and industrial engineer, President of Light Energy Company. "The best analogy for you is to understand it like a radio station. If you turn on a single station, your radio will...understand it, but if you turn on fifty different stations at once...you can't understand any of it. The cells in our body, turns out, have the same functionality."[109]

Biostimulation is a medical treatment that uses either a monochromatic or isolated range of light wavelengths, predominately infrared or red wavelengths of light. Biostimulation is also known as:

- light therapy
- biostimulation
- low intensity laser therapy (LILT)
- low level laser therapy (LLLT)
- cold laser therapy
- photobiological treatment
- photo-biomodulation
- photonic stimulation
- photo therapy

Light activates DNA, which then transmits this new energy to the cell walls by means of protein and calcium. The cell walls then transform into healthy shapes so the cell can perform normally once again and function at a higher capacity. The irradiated tissue activates nitric oxide, thus increasing blood flow that helps to carry vitamins and nutrients to lacking areas; likewise, toxins and metabolic by-products are taken away from the suffering

---

[109] Olszewski D., Interview - Seattle, Washington. (2001)

tissue quickly. Biostimulatory light therapy activates the stimulation, synthesis and production of:

- collagen
- nitric oxide
- ATP (adenosine triphosphate)
- elastin
- fibroblast activity

Unfortunately, the photobiological basis of biostimulation is not well understood, and the acceptance of light therapy has suffered as a result. Kendric Smith Emeritus, former Professor of Radiation Oncology at Stanford University School of Medicine, has been researching light's effects on healing since 1966. He notes when cells are underperforming or not growing well, exposing them to specific wavelengths encourages chemical and physical changes and spurs development, growth and activity. A long-time photobiology researcher, Smith believes ignorance about photobiology and photophysics is a major deterrent to the mainstream use of light medicine, even though it has been proved effective in several clinical situations.[110]

The United States Department of Defense (DOD) and DARPA (Defense Advanced Research Projects Agency) found post-op patients treated with light therapy needed fewer analgesics for pain.[111] They have developed a mobile light therapy device to accelerate healing on soldiers in the field. As Professor of Anatomy Physiology in the Genetics University of the Health Sciences Medical School, Juanita Anders Ph.D. has been part of the development process.[112] It is believed the technology stimulates growth factors beneficial for regeneration while decreasing the inflammatory response.

Federal Drug Administration (FDA) Center Engineer of Physics with Devices and Radiological Health, Offices of Science and Engineering Laboratories, Ronald Waynant expressed light has the potential to help build people's immune systems.[113] According to Waynant, this photobiological research has also shown damage from a heart attack or stroke can be reduced by fifty percent just by putting a powerful light device on the victim's head or

---

[110] Smith, K.C., Interview - Palo Alto, California. (2002)
[111] Waynant, R., Interview - San Jose, California. (2007)
[112] Anders, J., Interview - San Jose, California. (2007)
[113] Waynant, R., Anders, J., Rigau, J., Light Activated Tissue Regeneration & Therapy II. (2007)

chest shortly after the incident. He feels this technology has tremendous value to the nation and the world. With Anders he worked on a DOD project attempting to initiate super human strength in soldiers with specific wavelengths of light.

Nerve sprouting after trauma is an extremely slow process, and often, the damaged part of the body does not recover the same sensitivity or ability it once had. Dr. Shimon Rochkind, Department of Neurosurgery, Division of Peripheral Nerve Reconstruction, Tel Aviv University, has researched the applications of light therapy in clinical settings.[114] He is working with patients who are dealing with the effects of nerve injuries. Rochkind has found nerve sprouts regenerate at double the rate under red laser light, and full recovery is more likely.[115]

In many cases, traditional medicine masks or suppresses symptoms rather than restores the cell to normal function. "Light therapy does not just manage the pain but gets rid of it by curing the problem," said Fred Kahn, M.D. President of Meditech International, manufacturer of the Bioflex light therapy device. As a last resort, after traditional therapies had failed, patients found relief and recovery through light therapy. On a regular basis, his technology has helped avert amputation on people with severe diabetic lesions. His objective is to return patients to a normal state of health with as few drugs as possible.[116] Insurance companies are now adopting this medical treatment because they are finding it saves money. With CPT (current procedural terminology) codes for light therapy treatments now in use by the American Medical Association, light therapy is now a viable and economical treatment option to insurance companies.

Before developing his light therapy devices, Kahn spent several years of research consulting closely with many prominent scientists, including Dr. Mary Dyson, Emeritus Professor of Physiology, University of London and Dr. Tiina Karu, Professor of Laser Biology and Medicine at the Russian Academy of Science in Moscow. According to Karu (one of the first scientists in the world to publish controlled studies of the effects of biostimulation on cells), "The language of the cells is light. We can talk to cells with light. We just don't know their language."

---

[114] Rochkind, S., Interview - Toronto, Canada. (2006)
[115] Rochkind, S., Phototherapy in peripheral nerve injury for muscle preservation and nerve regeneration. (2009)
[116] Kahn, F., Interview - Toronto, Canada. Low intensity laser therapy in clinical practice. (2006)

As mentioned in Chapter two, the Russians were early leaders in light technology. They conducted numerous studies documenting positive results on medical conditions, such as:

- intestinal ulcers
- bronchial asthma
- pulmonary tuberculosis
- lung disease
- thrombosis
- head trauma
- maxillary sinusitis
- chronic tonsillitis
- cysts
- cardiac arteries conditions
- heart disease
- dermatological ulcers
- burns
- traumas
- pneumonia
- autoimmune
- diabetes
- gynecological issues

In the United Kingdom, James Carroll, founder of Thor Photomedicine Ltd., began manufacturing biostimulation equipment for treating animals, including the Queen of England's horse. Carroll now has medical approvals to treat humans for pain management of arthritis, back and neck pain, inflammatory conditions, and asthma. Carroll sees biostimulation eventually in every hospital department, and ultimately ending up in the medicine cabinet of every home. "Over 1000 papers have been published...Credibility is critical for acceptance by reimbursement and regulatory authorities, doctors, and therapists," said Carroll.[117]

Another advocate of using light therapy on animals is Deborah Carroll, Director of Rehabilitation and Conditioning at Central Texas Veterinary Specialty Hospital, a certified Canine Rehabilitation Practitioner and NSCA Conditioning Specialist. She began using laser and LED devices

---

[117] Carroll, J., Interview - San Jose, California. (2007)

in 2005 on animals for various indications, including neurological and degenerative disease, injuries and other issues. Carroll has a protocol combining the laser with other traditional treatments. She is able to heal animals quickly with minimal scarring, especially in post surgical wounds.[118]

An article in *Neuroscience* in June of 2008, addressing photobiological experiments performed at the Department of Neurobiology Medical College of Wisconsin, suggested that infrared LED therapy may be valuable in the treatment of damaged neurons caused by Parkinson's disease.[119] Indeed, some research indicates biostimulation can be used to halt the effects of Alzheimer's disease. Light not only passes through skin and muscle tissue, but also through bones, including the skull, thus allowing it to treat problems with the brain. Researchers noted that infrared treatments (infrared helmets worn for ten minutes each day) had positive effects on Alzheimer's patients' cognitive function and learning performance. Not only did the treatments slow the progress of the disease, but in some cases, they partially restored cognitive functioning that had already been lost.[120]

Light therapy devices have proved successful in sports medicine. MedX developed equipment using lasers and super luminous light emitting diodes within the same device console. When talking with V.P. of Scientific Affairs of MedX Anita Saltmarche explained even though she sees resistance to light therapy in the medical community, she believes consumers will ultimately drive this technology into the market place.

Saltmarche also believes this technology is barely scratching the surface of its potential. MedX lights are used in sports medicine by professional franchises, including the Boston Celtics and the San Jose Sharks.[121] A professional athlete may be treated three times a day to accelerate healing and keep pain under control, and will usually see a significant decrease in pain and swelling after a few treatments. It is not unusual to have six to eight treatments, and chronic conditions may need twelve to twenty. Arthritic patients may get standard monthly treatments to keep pain under control.

---

[118] Carroll, D., Interview - Austin, Texas. (2010)
[119] Liang H.L., Whelan H.T., Eells J.T., Wong-Riley M.T. Near-infrared light via light-emitting diode treatment is therapeutic against rotenone- and 1-methyl-4-phenylpyridinium ion-induced neurotoxicity. (2008)
[120] http://news.injuryboard.com/alzheimer39s-helmet-may-send-healing-light-to-brain.aspx?googleid=29284 (2008)
[121] Saltmarche, A., Interview - San Jose, California. (2007)

Several professional athletes and sports franchises, including the NFL, NBL and the NBA, are utilizing Meditech International equipment. Dr. Kenneth Mikkelsen, the chiropractor for the Canadian Olympic swim team uses state of the art equipment in his clinics. After seeking different modalities of treatment, he discovered light therapy. While continuously seeking ways to enhance the performance of athletes, he experienced high rates of success with light in treating difficult cases. Within weeks of introducing two Meditech systems, the results were so significant Mikkelsen purchased two more, stating, "I have added a whole new level of care."[122]

Due to constant joint stress, many of the athletes suffer from arthritis. Light therapy alleviated their symptoms. Chuck Mooney, an athletic therapist for the Toronto Raptors, began using the Meditech International system on players with recurring lower back issues; his patients saw immediate results. Inspired by the rapid healing, Mooney tried the process on a player's ankle injury, which also yielded rapid recovery.[123]

Chiropractor Dr. Leonard Rudnick said, "It's not about treating symptoms...This is about returning cells to normal function." In many cases, Rudnick's more skeptical patients were referred to him by relatives or friends pressuring them into trying light treatment. Skeptics are his favorite patients because, "When they get better, they know it is not the placebo effect." For good results, Rudnick says it is best to use red first and infrared wavelength second. He has worked with many commercial photobiological therapy devices and observed a considerable drop in effectiveness with devices when both wavelengths are used simultaneously.[124]

Chukuka Enwemeka, Ph.D. and Dean of the New York Institute of Technology looked at the repair process of tendons. He found not only laser treatment could enhance the healing process of tendons but discovered lasers were also beneficial to tissue repair. As a doctoral student, he recognized one of the most beneficial areas of light therapy is resolving inflammation and swelling. Light therapy is also effective on non-healing wounds and stubborn fractures. "We are talking about a therapy that will get a patient better; it costs significantly less money, and upon recovering, the person becomes an active contributor to society as opposed to being a dependent," he said.

---

[122] Mikkelsen, K., Interview - Toronto, Canada. (2006)
[123] Mooney, C., Interview - Toronto, Canada. (2006)
[124] Rudnick, L., Interview - Toronto, Canada. (2006)

Enwemeka revealed carpal tunnel syndrome is reversed by applying light, typically within eight to twelve treatments. The cost for a carpal tunnel treatment is about $1500 using light therapy. The cost of surgery is about $25,000. Enwemeka feels the first step to healing an injury should be with the use of light. His research also explores diabetic lesions. In severe cases patients end up losing legs and limbs. When serious skin ulcers are treated with light, over fifty percent respond positively with complete healing. "It may seem low, but these are limbs that would have been amputated. That's a great saving!"   There are also many cases of eliminating addicting pain medications, antibiotics, and pain, which allows people to get back to work. "We are looking at billions and billions of dollars that could be saved by doing something as simple as treating diabetic ulcer patients with light," said Dr. Enwemeka.[125]

Current methods of treatment for chronic diabetic ulcers costs about $45,000 per patient annually. With millions of people inflicted, the costs add up. In January of 2004, *Diabetes Care Journal* published a double-blind study about treating diabetic lesions with monochromatic infrared light. The twenty-seven person study used the Anodyne equipment, with very encouraging results.[126] It has been found while a small percentage of people do not respond to light therapy, others respond very quickly. More research needs to be done, but it is plausible this problem is connected to vitamin, mineral, enzyme deficiency, environmental toxin. Could low systemic levels of nitric oxide be a major factor? According to Nathan S. Bryan, Ph.D. Professor of Molecular Medicine at the University of Texas, and Co-Founder Neogenis Labs, "something unsuspecting such as mouthwash can deplete nitric oxide from the body in moments."[127]

Photobiological laser therapy is also being used for dental problems. Dr. Diane Mediguzzo, a dentist working out of the University of Sao Paulo, Brazil, has been treating patients with periodontal (gum) disease using laser technology where a fiber optic cable is inserted into each pocket between the teeth; the pockets are then sterilized by a laser. So far Dr. Mediguzzo has had

---

[125] Enwemeka, C., Interview - Toronto, Canada. (2006)
[126] Leonard, D.R., Farooqi, M.H., and Myers, S. Restoration of Sensation, Reduced Pain, and Improved Balance in Subjects With Diabetic Peripheral Neuropathy: A double-blind, randomized, placebo-controlled study with monochromatic near-infrared treatment. (2004)
[127] Bryan, S. Nathan, Zand, Janet, Gottlieb, Bill, - The Nitric Oxide (NO) Solution. (2010)

an eighty percent success rate, and the treatment works faster and is more affordable than traditional dental treatments. It is very effective in eliminating periodontal disease, while giving a secondary biostimulatory healing effect. Patients' gums heal much faster and there is less chance of the periodontal disease returning. Dental Technologies in the United States is treating patients with similar technology. Brazilians are experimenting with a new technology that treats periodontal disease using a photodynamic drug applied to the gums. After the sensitizer is absorbed, the gums are exposed to light.[128] Millenium Dental Technologies, Inc. uses the PerioLase®, a similar technology to eradicate gum disease.

Using low wattage lasers reduces the need for pain analgesics with patients. Since 1989, Arun A. Darbar, D.D.S., has been successfully using lasers to manage pain in dental, cosmetic and reconstructive dentistry.[129] Currently Darbar uses lasers for both surgery and accelerated healing. He has had great success with dental cysts and in regenerating bone tissue in periodontal pockets. Using lasers helps patients avoid expensive and painful periodontal surgery as well. In cases where invasive surgery is inevitable, using laser surgical equipment speeds up the healing process significantly, due partially to its secondary biostimulatory effect. Furthermore, Darbar successfully uses laser therapy to treat oral ulcers (mouth sores), especially in patients with braces.

Paul Bradley, D.D.S., has also been using lasers to help dental surgery patients heal faster. Bradley specializes in dental surgery but is always looking for less invasive procedures to treat his patients. Learning about lasers changed his practice, and it became apparent that using hot lasers in surgical procedures has a secondary low intensity biostimulatory effect on tissue that reduced pain and sped up the recovery process.[130]

The cover story of the January 2001 issue of *National Geographic*, "The Body in Space," featured the use of high-output LEDs to stimulate the organelles which promote healing.[131] NASA has been using biostimulation technology in space missions since 2000, according to Weijia Zhou, Ph.D., Director of the Wisconsin Center for Space Automation and Robotics at the University of Wisconsin. NASA has also discovered that plants only need two specific light wavelengths to grow and mature; one which falls in the red

---

[128] Mediguzzo, D., Interview - San Jose, California. (2007)
[129] Darbar, A.A., Interview - Toronto, Canada. (2006)
[130] Bradley, P., Interview - Toronto, Canada. (2006)
[131] Whelan, H.T., The Body in Space. (2001)

area of the spectrum and the second in the area perceived as blue.[132] Dr. Harry T. Whelan of Milwaukee, Wisconsin was issued one of the early FDA approvals for photobiological devices to be used with patients. Working with NASA and Quantum Devices, Inc., he is taking large steps in this new field and has had overwhelming success treating patients with brain tumors and many other ailments.[133]

Technology Transfer Office at Marshall Space Flight Center in Huntsville, Alabama, NASA is developing high output LEDs with heat-sinks permitting a greater volume of light. Some of their arrays emit light brighter than the sun; when illuminating cultured cells from the newly developed LEDs, scientist were able to grow muscle cells at a much faster speed than would be possible under normal conditions. Donald J. Stillwell is responsible for cultivating new medical technology at NASA and developing practical applications for photobiological treatments.

The United States Navy also uses biostimulation with their Special Forces and on submarines. Prolonged weightlessness in space prevents the healing of even the smallest cut or injury; in many cases wounds do not heal up until the astronaut is back on Earth. In space, the cells' mitochondria do not function properly. Irradiating tissue with biostimulation triggers a biochemical reaction that stabilizes cell function. When LED light therapy is used, astronauts in space are able to recover.

Len Saputo, M.D. of the Health Medicine Institute (HMI) in Walnut Creek, California has been treating patients with infrared light for over ten years. Patients with injuries, chronic pain and other ailments have benefited, in many cases alleviating their need for drugs and pain medication. "The only way to turn this system around is to reverse our thinking and start looking at personal health measures to prevent disease." Saputo is an advocate of Complementary Alternative Medicine (CAM), and his book, *A Return to Healing: Radical Health Care Reform and the Future of Medicine*, exposes a broken medical system that is doing its best to keep the status-quo. Saputo points out how corporatized medicine only gets to work once disease occurs. Saputo believes non-invasive treatments should be a first line of defense and

[132] Zhou, W., Interview second unit production, Mile Newcomb - Madison, Wisconsin. (2001)
[133] Schmidt, M.H., Reichert K.W., Ozker K., Meyer G.A., Donohoe D.L., Bajic D.M., Whelan N.T., Whelan H.T. Preclinical evaluation of benzoporphyrin derivative combined with a light-emitting diode array for photodynamic therapy of brain tumors Pediatric Neurosurgery. (1999)

feels the integrative-medical approach is the future of medicine (traditional and alternative together).[134]

Brian Hulbert of LuxWaves™ Inc. says, "light technology will revolutionize medicine. It is a cost effective alternative to drugs and surgery...using a light therapy device in conjunction with amino acid supplements hyper-accelerates the healing response. LuxWaves Inc. is the only company in the world offering nitric oxide activators with light." This technology has the ability to reduce pain drug intake and the need for anti-inflammatory medications.

There are some incidents where biostimulation can cause secondary occurrences or side effects, but not in the traditional sense; these are actually positive side effects. A few side effects Rudnick witnessed occurred when he used light therapy on a patient suffering carpal tunnel syndrome.[135] The patient's blood sugar had been regularly in the 400 range. When visiting his regular doctor, it was discovered that his blood sugar had dropped down to 110. When the doctor asked him what he had been doing differently, the patient replied that there was nothing out of the ordinary. When pressed further, he suddenly remembered he had been receiving light therapy.

This is not the only case of positive side effects. Another case involved a patient with an injured wrist; after several treatments with light, the patient's fibromyalgia symptoms were significantly reduced.

Yet another patient suffering low back pain was treated with light around the abdominal region with a secondary effect in that the patient's Crohn's disease was relieved. Rudnick's reputation is drawing clients all over the world to visit him in Tucson, Arizona, and he touts a success rate of over ninety percent in patients treated with light.

In one instance, a patient was undergoing therapy for facial wrinkles with a red/infrared APL device. After several treatments, she began experiencing vision problems. She wore permanent contact lenses, and feeling concerned, she immediately contacted her optometrist. In the meantime, she also contacted her light therapist, believing her vision problems were a direct result of the light treatments. The light therapist, however, was adamant about the fact that light only heals cells, never damages them. Eventually the optometrist confirmed this. Upon removing

---

[134] Saputo, Len, M.D. and Belitsos, Byron, A Return to Healing: Radical Health Care Reform and the Future of Medicine. (2009)
[135] Rudnick, L., Interview - Toronto, Canada. (2006)

her contacts lenses, the optometrist discovered that the patient's vision had definitely changed— her vision had improved! Now she needed a weaker prescription. This beneficial secondary effect is rarely seen within the medical community. Even the use of high wattage hot lasers in surgery has a secondary healing effect because of the lower level of light radiation also being emitted.[136]

Likewise, dentists have found significantly less infection when using lasers, compared to using traditional scalpel incisions.[137] Dentists have now discovered that lowering the wattage on surgical lasers speeds up the recovery time and reduces the risk of infection.

Light therapy continually proves effective in treating a wide array of medical conditions. In addition, these biostimulatory therapies do not have the negative side effects associated with traditional surgical or pharmaceutical treatments. Rather, doctors and practitioners are noticing that light therapies do tend to have additional positive after effects. It has been discovered when patients undergo light treatment for one condition, they find other problems have resolved, changed or healed.

While the Russians, Europeans, Japanese and Middle Easterners have not been shy to forge ahead in this new science, to date, the FDA has approved only a relatively limited number of biostimulation devices. Despite FDA resistance, American scientists continue to publish more papers confirming photobiological proof that light indeed heals.

PHOTODYNAMIC THERAPY

Photodynamic therapy (PDT) is photochemical destruction of diseased tissue. PDT eliminates cancer, tumors or irregular cells from proliferating without damaging the surrounding cells. The mechanism of a photodynamic treatment is made up of two primary components: a chemical compound that induces light sensitivity in cell tissue and either a laser or high powered LED device applied to affected area.

These light-activated drugs are injected or applied topically. A topical photosensitizer called aminolevulinic acid (ALA) is used to treat skin cancer. The injected photosensitizer (commonly Photofrin or Radachlorin) saturates and accumulates in all of the abnormal or cancerous tissue. The fast-growing

---

[136] Darbar. A., Interview - Toronto, Canada. (2006)
[137] Bradley, P., Interview - Toronto, Canada. (2006)

cancerous cells absorb the photosensitive dye much more readily than normal tissue. The patient waits twenty-four to forty-eight hours to allow the chemical to exit the healthy tissue, while the drug accumulates in the cancer or problem cells. The light device is then applied to the affected areas. In cases targeting internal organs, a fiber optic cable is connected to an endoscope or bronchial scope. Once the light is applied, the treatment can be completed in a short amount of time. "The appeal of photodynamic therapy is that rather than using cold surgical steel to create a scar and stitches on the skin, we are giving a drug and then shining light on the skin," said Professor Harvey Luis, M.D., of the University of British Columbia.

The FDA approval of PDT is a difficult process. Richard Felton, a senior FDA official, explains, "What we have is a combination drug and device system…The difference is that in photodynamic therapy, you have to have both a drug and a light system to provide a clinical benefit." In other words, there are two different departments working together to analyze the data thus making this type of approval more complicated.

Overall, PDT is completed without painful surgery, chemotherapy or radiation, thereby avoiding the side effects and long healing time of traditional treatments. The only known side effects of PDT is a tendency to sunburn easily, which can be avoided by staying out of direct sunlight for several days or weeks afterwards, depending on treatment. Professor Stephen Bown M.D. of the University College Medical School in London sums up PDT as such: "Photodynamic therapy is new technique for localizing an area for tissue destruction, but doing it in a gentle way so the natural body mechanisms will clean things up afterwards, so patients don't require any radical intervention such as surgery. It has the other added advantage that if you miss a bit, you can go back and do it again. For surgery and radiation treatments, that is a lot more difficult."[138]

Drugs that will reduce the time of light sensitivity are currently in developmental stages. Successful medical treatment of cancer with porphyrins (light sensitive molecules) was first developed by Dr. Thomas Dougherty of Roswell Park Cancer Research Institute in New York City. In 1973, Dougherty successfully eradicated tumor cells using a light sensitive

---

[138] Bown, S.G., Interview - Vancouver, Canada. (2001)

compound and a slide projector. His motivation, persistence and self-funded research made photodynamic therapy what it is today.[139]

Richard Whyte, M.D. of Stanford University says that clinical trials are being conducted to test the effectiveness of PDT on breast cancer. These studies suggest that PDT may be more effective than standard laser therapies because light penetrates deeper into tissue, resulting in a prolonged effect that prevents the re-growth of tumors.[140]

Another professor researching PDT treatment, Michael Hamblin Ph.D. of Harvard Medical School, believes the combination of PDT with certain immunostimulants can produce highly synergistic benefits, including the regression of distant untreated tumors. He is looking at how PDT can activate the host immune system to attack more advanced stages of cancer.

Sandra Gollnick, Ph.D. at Roswell Park Cancer Institute points to the same conclusion: "PDT is unique in its ability not just to treat cancer, but to create an immune response that prevents a recurrence."[141] The current treatment methods of surgery and chemotherapy eliminate cancer, but also weaken a patient's immune system. PDT exposes and destroys tumors without having an adverse effect on the rest of the body; furthermore, it exposes tumor antigens, triggering a response that vaccinates the patient. Gollnick believes there is potential in developing anti-cancer vaccines from this technology.

UC Davis Medical Center in Sacramento, California has early technology adopters treating patients with PDT. Ronald Hsu M.D. has been successful in treating esophagus cancer and Roblee Allen, M.D. treated lung cancer with this technology. Allen was involved with early trials using photodynamic drugs and said, "It doesn't matter how you generate the light as long as you deliver the appropriate wavelength to stimulate the drug; it's a photo toxic effect to kill the diseased cells."[142]

Allen mentioned how light sensitive drugs can also be used to detect tumors not visible to the naked eye. "So we can use it in both the diagnostic and therapeutic sense." Photobiological research on using PDT for diagnosing disease is being conducted in Tennessee. Dr. Bergein Overholt of the Thompson Cancer Survival Center has focused on this research, which

---

[139] Dougherty, T.J., A brief history of clinical photodynamic therapy development at Roswell Park Cancer Institute. (1996)
[140] Whyte, R., Interview - Stanford, California. (2002)
[141] Gollnick, S., Interview - Vancouver, Canada. (2001)
[142] Hsu, R., M.D., Interview - Davis, California. (2001)

will allow for cancer diagnoses without invasive surgery. The procedure, known as optical biopsy, is much more efficient than standard biopsy. "Eight optical biopsies can be done in the time it takes for one standard procedure, at a fraction of the cost," said Overholt.

Light sensitive porphyrins are not only used for diagnosis and cancer eradication, but also for the treatment of arterial diseases. In arterial disease, arteries are blocked by fatty deposits or plaque, limiting proper circulation and leading to a number of health issues. While surgical procedures such as angioplasty are available, they are invasive, and often, the disease will return.

Professor Bown has been developing a light therapy system in order to melt away arterial plaque. He said, "One of those most exciting programs we have going on at the moment is using PDT in arterial diseases. Now arterial diseases are the biggest killer in Western countries because arteries get partially or completely blocked by fatty deposits." It is difficult to perform surgical procedure on the peripheral arteries, arteries in the leg, neck or arteries in the heart. In contrast, with light therapy a thin balloon is introduced into the artery, and then inflated. An optical fiber slides into the area and the laser is activated. It is typically a simple ten minute treatment causing few complications. Bown is also looking at PDT for treating cancers in two other areas. "We have been working on using PDT for cancers in the prostate and the pancreas. The laser fibers go directly into the gland to deliver light to destroy the cancerous area."[143]

PDT is also useful for the photobiological treatment of macular degeneration, a leading cause of blindness. There are two types of macular degeneration: the dry type, in which the macula (the pigmented layer under the retina) deteriorates, and the wet type, in which blood vessels break through the deteriorated macula, bleed and scar. While traditional laser treatment is sometimes a useful therapy for wet macular degeneration, it is a risky procedure and often not appropriate for advanced cases. Dr. Daniel Brinton explains how photodynamic therapy is less risky than laser therapy, because it does not run the risk of causing burns or further damage to the eye.[144] After injecting photosynthetic dye, light is applied, and when the dye reacts, it destroys the leaking vessels. While these treatments are not able to improve any vision lost in macular degeneration, it does keep the disease

---

[143] Bown S. G., Interview - Vancouver, Canada. (2001)
[144] Brinton, D., Interview - Oakland, California. (2003)

from progressing, and patients tend to have stable vision with occasional retreatment.

Hamblin is a prolific leader in applications of photo-medicine in both of the fields PDT and biostimulation and has published over 100 peer-reviewed articles. His book, *Advances in Photodynamic Therapy,* is one of the most comprehensive texts on PDT in the field.[145] "I think that one of the biggest applications for this is the worldwide rise in multi-antibiotic resistant infections. Suddenly the World Health Organization has decided that it is a major health problem. A person could check into a hospital and have surgical wounds infected with bacteria for which there are no available antibiotics — there is great interest in being able to treat infections with means other than antibiotics, and photodynamic therapy may be one of these," he suggested.

In experimental testing, Hamblin induces infection by placing bacteria into a wound. Then he applies photosensitizer to the wound, allowing it to bind with the bacteria. After the photosensitizer penetrates the bacteria, a light is focused on the treatment area. Hamblin points out, "With bacteria such as e-coli, which are responsible for many wound infections, the infection goes away as you shine the light. Within a half hour the bacteria are gone; their wounds heal perfectly well after you have treated them."

In cases with a more invasive bacterium, a common problem for burn patients, Hamblin found when burns are treated, not only is the infection cured, but the wounds also heal significantly faster than when treated with other traditional anti-bacterial agents. He concludes that PDT may not only destroy the bacteria, but it may also destroy the enzymes, toxins and other virulent factors the bacteria produce which slow down wound healing.

Hamblin believes PDT could be used for other localized infections in the stomach and lungs. "A possible future application could be with patients who have cystic fibrosis, who are very susceptible to bacterial infection. Envision an aerosol mist containing a photosensitizer that patients breathe in. How best to deliver the light? One [way] is by placing the light source through a bronchoscope, but the infection tends to be diffused. The second is to use a very bright red light and go right through the chest, because red light travels through tissue...gets through the lungs damaging the bacteria. Both those options would have to be explored in later studies," stated Hamblin.

---

[145] Hamblin, M.R., Interview - Vancouver, Canada. (2001)

Helicobacter pylori are a bacterium that lives under the mucus layer of the stomach and causes both ulcers and stomach cancer. It is the most common infection in the world. The treatment is a complicated course of triple antibiotic therapy. A certain number of patients do not respond to the antibiotics because the bacterium has become resistant. According to Hamblin, "It's possible you could just drink the photosensitizer and the light would be delivered through a normal endoscope to the stomach and beamed over the stomach wall, and hopefully the bacteria would be eradicated. This is also something to really study in the future."

Reports about new strains of bacteria becoming antibiotic resistant are rising, inspiring a frantic research effort in the pharmaceutical industry, which spends millions of dollars to discover new antibiotic products. Hamblin believes there are readily available inexpensive photosensitizers and light sources to which bacteria will never develop a resistance.

Another medical problem that could be treated with light therapy is called necrotizing fasciitis, known as the "flesh-eating disease." This bacteria attacks so quickly that one could literally lose an arm within twelve hours; the bacterial infection simply races through the tissue. Existing treatment is by surgical incision, so if a limb is infected, it will have to be amputated. Hamblin believes it is possible to spray the photosensitizers onto the tissue and irradiate with light, halting the bacteria. While, there would still be much tissue damage, the limb perhaps could be saved.

Wolfgang Neuberger Ph.D., CEO of Biolitec AG in Jena, Germany, began making fiber optics equipment for various treatments in 1988, introducing some of the first lasers for PDT. After finding success with light delivery systems, he decided to develop PDT drugs. His company focuses on developing new, innovative drugs for the treatment of a broad range of diseases.

"We have fiber optic delivery systems and we've got photodynamic drugs so this enables us to easily customize these components for one optimal treatment," said Neuberger.

Temoporfin, a light sensitive drug to reduce inflammation of rheumatoid arthritis is one of the formulas developed by Biolitic AG. Neuberger is not shy about saying, "We are one of the pioneers in the medical laser field."

Biolitec AG has licensed many innovative formulas, enhancing drug selectivity for the treatment of many diseases, such as:

- mascular degeneration
- esophagus cancer
- prostate cancer
- skin cancer
- periodontal disease
- rheumatoid arthritis
- heart disease

Biolitec AG has been purchasing companies, creating synergistic alliances to further this technology and expand their market share in this relatively new field of photobiological science. "This translates to reduced treatment time for our drugs used in PDT to treat disease, making the method even more practicable and less expensive," says Neuberger.[146]

An important driving force in the field of photodynamic medicine is the International Photodynamic Association (IPA) based in Vancouver, British Columbia. "It's the coming together of science, industry, medical practitioners and government all in one setting to thrash out key issues as it relates to treating patients with light," said Dr. Harvey Lui, a dermatologist and former Chairman of IPA.[147] He said providing a forum of open communication and discussion is important because each scientist or physician has their own unique set of patient problems. Governments have issues about whether any new treatment is safe for the public; then industry has its issues and agendas to ensure it develops a commercially viable treatment, while still being responsible to share holders. So, each group has its unique vested interest to come together and the IPA platform facilitates it. One advantage of the photodynamic community is they are extremely open, compared to the competitive egos which seem rampant within other biomedical fields, according to Lui.

There is a powerful synergistic effect between the use of light and drugs together. Combining these two technologies opens up a number of possibilities for potential innovation and growth.

---

[146] Neuberger, W., Interview - Vancouver, Canada. (2001)
[147] Lui, H., Interview - Vancouver, Canada. (2001)

BLOOD IRRADIATION

Blood Irradiation (BI) works by triggering a photochemical reaction that cleans and revitalizes the blood, accelerating the healing process within the entire body. The device systems and methods used to execute treatment can be very different. There are two common wavelengths of light primary used, UV and red, each responsible for different biochemical actions. Both wavelengths have a positive systemic effect on the body.

In his 2003 book, *Close-to-Nature Medicine,* Kenneth Dillon, Ph.D. clearly points out the overwhelming data proving light has the ability to destroy pathogens in the blood.[148] "Human beings have a chemiluminescent immune system," he said.   He also points out blood irradiation is accomplished by utilizing the body's own natural defenses to recognize and annihilate the sick, diseased cells. Dillon said, "It is very shocking that, after 20 years of a devastating epidemic...the medical establishment has still failed to test this excellent therapy."

How much control do humans really have over stopping a global pandemic outbreak? The United States considers resistant infection a "very high priority," and so has created a coalition to eliminate the possible threat. The coalition is composed of the Center for Disease Control (CDC), Active Bacterial Core surveillance (ABCs), Emerging Infections Programs (EIP), Transatlantic Task Force on Antibiotic Resistance (TATFAR) and Infectious Diseases Society of America (IDSA).

The current belief is that there is no way to deal with a catastrophe of that scale. Multi drug-resistant bacteria have been around for decades. Bacteria are equipped with a gene enabling them to produce an enzyme that disables antibiotics, rendering the drugs powerless.[149]

The World Health Organization (WHO) has recommended countries around the world pay serious attention to the emergence of this resistance factor. The *Handbook of Biosurveillance,* published in 2006,[150] outlines principles that apply to both natural and man-made biowar epidemics. Bioterrorism is the intentional release or dissemination of biological agents into the environment to cause illness or death in people,

---

[148] Dillon, K., Close-to-Nature Medicine. (2003)
[149] Mckenna, M., Superbug: the Fatal Menace of MRSA. (2010)
[150] Wagner, M. M., Handbook of Bioserveillance. (2006)

animals, or plants. They include the use of germ bacterium, viruses, prions, fungal agents and biological toxins.

As disease resistance continues with current medications, and biowar threats loom in the distance, the need for reliable and effective alternative treatments becomes even greater. The use of light based medical technology may be the only viable solution as harmful bacterial and viral cells contain up to five times more photosensitive amino acids, making them extremely susceptible to destruction by light.

Blood irradiation using UV light is most commonly called ultraviolet blood irradiation (UBI). This treatment removes a small amount blood from the patient, exposes it to light then returns the blood back to the patient intravenously. This system is quite effective at removing harmful substances and has proven effective in:

- inactivating pathogens and contaminants
- destroying viruses
- eliminating bacteria
- inactivating toxins
- inactivating snake venom
- activating white blood cells
- helping blood viscosity acting as a blood thinner
- increasing blood oxygen transport
- decreasing platelet aggregation
- removing of fungi and parasites
- inactivating e-coli
- causing diphtheria to become unstable
- causing tetanus to become unstable
- helping vascular conditions and circulatory activities, improving circulation
- reducing arterial plaque
- decreasing swelling
- stabilizing alkalinity
- increasing intracellular antioxidants that buffer and neutralize free radicals
- balancing calcium and phosphorous
- accelerating the lymphatic system
- stimulating antibody production

- immunizing the body against disease
- activating steroid hormones
- producing a positive effect on the autonomic nervous system
- stimulating corticosteroid production
- helping to reduce nausea and vomiting
- reducing symptoms of candida
- reducing symptoms of chronic fatigue
- reducing symptoms of allergies
- reducing symptoms of emphysema
- reducing diabetic complications
- reducing symptoms of rheumatologic diseases
- helping to eliminate acute colds
- helping to eliminate flu
- reducing symptoms of fibromyalgia
- assisting in recovery of stroke
- reducing symptoms of bronchitis
- reducing chemical sensitivity
- helping reduce problem relating to arterial disease
- reducing symptoms of macular degeneration

Blood irradiation with light is a treatment system that has been reinvented several times throughout modern medical history, first by the Danish, then the Americans and more recently, the Russians. Strangely however, it has never taken hold, even with all its remarkable results. Blood Irradiation is known by many terms including:

- extracorporeal photopheresis
- ultraviolet blood irradiation (UBI)
- intravenous laser blood irradiation (ILBI)
- blood photomodifcation
- trans-dermal blood irradiation (TDBI)
- sublingual blood irradiation
- extracorporeal photochemotherapy
- photoluminescence therapy
- biophotonic therapy
- photobiological therapy
- hemo-irradiation phototherapy
- hematologic oxidative therapy

- ultraviolet hemo-irradiation phototherapy

An excerpt from the American Cancer Society's website reads, "A special form of UV blood irradiation called photopheresis...also inhibits T-cell lymphoma and may be helpful for other conditions. Proponents of UV blood irradiation claim UV...kills germs...inside the body and...neutralizes toxins in the blood. Some claim even a small amount of UV treated blood can reenter the circulatory system of the patient and stimulate the immune system...against invaders, including cancer cells." Ultraviolet blood irradiation treatment is approved by the FDA for treating T-cell lymphoma. Some clinical trial results look promising for the treatment of immune system diseases such as: [151]

- multiple sclerosis
- systemic sclerosis
- rheumatoid arthritis
- lupus
- type 1 diabetes

BI treatments have advanced since they were first developed. In some cases people are injected with light sensitive compounds prior to light exposure. There are other systems that remove the blood and then mix it with compounds followed by exposure to light. In other scenarios, hydrogen peroxide is mixed into the blood as it circulates, to increase oxygen in the blood. Here are a few methods to conduct this process:

- intravenously, wherein the blood is circulated for exposure in a closed loop system
- blood is drawn, put into a irradiation device, and then re-injected
- laser inside a needle inserted directly into vein
- trans-dermal, a high powered LED or low wattage laser is placed onto skin on specific location
- sublingually, placing the light under the tongue

---

[151]www.cancer.org/Treatment/TreatmentsandSideEffects/ComplementaryandAlternativeMedicine/ManualHealingandPhysicalTouch/light-therapy (2012)

In standard BI treatment, a patient is taken through the following process: The amount of blood irradiated during the treatment depends upon a patient's body weight. This is based upon a ratio of approximately 1/16th of the patient's blood. In some cases an anticoagulant such as Heparin is added to prevent the blood from clotting. The treatment begins when a needle is placed into the arm which is connected to a UV recirculation system. The patient's blood is drawn and then placed into a device where the syringe rotates slowly for a few minutes, exposing the blood to UV light. The irradiated blood is then injected back into the patient.

Sessions for either photobiological treatment take about an hour and can be done two to three times per week for several weeks, depending upon the severity of the disease. In the most severe cases, patients can receive treatment as often as once every twenty-four hours; less severe cases require fewer treatments.

In Denmark at the beginning twentieth century, Finsen developed a quasi-UV light system using a prism. As a victim of Pick's Disease, he noticed spending time in the sun alleviated some of his conditions such as anemia and fatigue. When available literature could not help him explain the change, he began researching the lights' power. Soon after, Walter Ude reported success in treating several cases of acute streptococcal infection by irradiating the skin with UV light, emulating Finsen's innovations.[152]

Then in 1928 Emmit S. Knott developed equipment to perform the BI process intravenously.[153] Knott pioneered blood irradiation on dogs before treating humans. His first patient suffered from a bacterial blood infection (sepsis), but recovered rapidly after the treatment. Knott, while working with Dr. Virgil Hancock, had great results and published their findings in 1934. By 1942 they had treated over 6,500 patients. During that era, Dr. George Miley, a clinical professor at Hahnemann Hospital and College of Medicine in Philadelphia, reported 151 consecutive cases with astounding results when patients were treated with UBI. Miley, however, noted a decrease in blood oxygen in many diseased states. The body consumes approximately 100 times more oxygen when it is responding to infection. Miley said there was a "pinking-up" of the patient's skin after treatment and a rise in blood oxygen levels without a rise in hemoglobin or red-cell count. In moderately advanced cases, ninety-eight percent recovered.

---

[152] Douglas, W.C., Into The Light. (1993)
[153] Knott, E., Development of Ultraviolet Blood Irradiation. (1948)

Miley treated a woman who had slipped into a coma from an almost certainly fatal infection brought on by botulism. Within seventy-two hours of her first UBI treatment, the woman was awake and mentally clear and was discharged thirteen days later.

American medical literature during the 1930s and early 1940s reported cases where dying patients responded to UBI treatment almost instantaneously, some within hours. In his 1943 book, *Ultraviolet Blood Irradiation*, Miley published the successful results of treating many diseases, including viral pneumonia. He noted that a complete disappearance of major symptoms occurred within twenty-four to seventy-two hours after a single UBI treatment. Coughing eased in three to seven days, and lungs cleared in one to four days. There is currently no other treatment available that produces such results.

In 1967 Robert Olney published material entitled *Blocked Oxidation* in which he pointed out cancer was a result of blocked oxidation within cells.[154] The data presented five cases of various cancers that were cured by a combination of techniques including UBI. Olney also treated individuals with hepatitis using UV light, documenting a study of forty-three patients with an average number of three treatments conducted on each.: Twenty-seven patients showed rapid reduction of symptoms, eleven showed marked improvement in four to seven days, and five showed improvement in eight to fourteen days. Dr. William Douglass has written several articles and books on health and medicine, and continues to uncover truths, while debunking deceptions within the medical community. He examines case studies and the mechanisms behind UBI and it near-miraculous results in his book, *Into the Light-Tomorrow's Medicine Today.*[155]

While most doctors focus on treating diseases, some like Len Saputo focus on wellness. Another proponent of wellness philosophy is Francisco Contreras, M.D. He examines patients holistically and analyzes all systemic and environmental factors. In his approach to medicine (conventional-alternative) he augments the best of both worlds. People from all over the world seek treatment at his Oasis of Hope Hospitals in California and Mexico.

There is a clear need to integrate this therapy into cancer treatment regimens, as they do not compromise the immune system or health of the

---

[154] Olney, R., Blocked Oxidation. (1967)
[155] Douglas, W. C., Into the Light: Tomorrow's Medicine Today! (2003)

patients.[156] Contreras mentions how effective UBI is in the treatment of hepatitis and pneumonia in his book, *Dismantling Cancer.* Some treatments include MOP-8. UV light destroys bacterial and viral pathogens and once the treated blood is back in the body, those dead pathogens produce a systemic "vaccination" effect and also act as antitumor agents. Additionally, the blood returned to the body continues to kill bacteria, viruses and toxins, and creates more white blood cells to resolve any systemic problems. How this mechanism works is not clearly understood, but according to Contreras, the blood holds radiation from its exposure to UV rays, and once back in the body, stimulates additional biochemical and photobiological reactions.

Incorporating light-activating agents such as MOP-8 increase the photobiological effect. Dr. Richard Edelson of Yale University developed a technique called UV extracorporeal photophoresis. The treatment requires separation of the white blood cells, which means UV light does not irradiate all of the blood. Unfortunately, there are many elements other than white blood cells that are photosensitive including:

- porphyrins
- antibodies
- steroids
- amino acids
- insulin
- liposomes

Some believe these elements should also be exposed to the light. In Edelson's technique the patient receives MOP-8 two hours before the blood is withdrawn. This therapy has proven successful and received FDA approval for the treatment of lymphoma; however, it costs several times more than traditional BI treatment.[157]

Another innovative method of treatment is a non-invasive system called sublingual UV photo-luminescent therapy where a device is placed under the tongue and the patient is irradiated with UV light for approximately an hour. This particular placement is effective since a tremendous amount of blood travels through the tongue. Thomas Perez,

---

[156] Contreras, F., Dismantling Cancer. (2005)
[157] Edelson R., Berger C., Gasparro F., et al. Treatment of cutaneous T-cell lymphoma by extracorporeal photochemotherapy. Preliminary results. (1987)

President of Harris Medical Resources, developed and successfully tested this new UBI treatment. His team testing in Africa obtained impressive preliminary results on twenty people infected with HIV. The largest expense during the clinical trials was the viral load tests. The cost of operating the light device is minimal. The patients received approximately forty one-hour treatments. A few patients felt so good afterwards that they left the study believing they were cured. Later, the majority of people were once again tested to determine viral load counts. According to Perez, there was no detectable level of HIV in the patient's blood.[158] This does not mean that the virus was completely gone, but it definitely was not in their blood, which is significant, because if the virus is not present, it cannot create symptoms.

There are few companies marketing UBI products. Longevity Resources Inc., a Canadian based company, calls their unit the Aquatron UV, manufactured in Germany. Touting it as reliable and extremely easy to use, this UV light is at a precise wavelength of 254nm. The practitioner buys sterile, single use disposable cuvettes made of high quality quartz glass. The duel UVC or UVA devices are double sided exposure systems. Another system marketed by Lumen Associates, a Canadian company, uses disposable materials to reduce costs and improve safety. President Doug Kemp believes his new system will provide quick, effective treatment and at a lower cost, compared to traditional UBI treatment. It treats blood via a syringe, in which it is drawn and exposed to UV light and then returned to the patient, thus eliminating the cuvette.

Other astounding results in the field of medical light are coming from Russian scientists and doctors. Years ago, the Russian medical system was funded by the former USSR government, so it was in their best interest to heal people quickly and inexpensively. This model forced innovations in health technology. The Russians developed a different clinical process of BI. They expanded the scope of BI by using lasers intravenously, calling it "intravenous laser blood irradiation" (ILBI). It was determined that the light's primary absorption point is the porphyrin (light sensitive) molecule, which creates a physicochemical chain reaction and activates an antioxidant defense system, which in turn, revitalizes the circulating cell population of neutrophils and makes them more resistant.

Great results have been reported by doctors; but, "the mechanism of it is not clear, yet scientists believe it is some sort of immune modulation,"

---

[158] Perez, T. - Phone Interview. (2007)

said Dr. Karu. When blood is irradiated during surgery, the blood becomes brighter, more oxygenated, and its viscosity lowers, becoming thinner and thus enabling better circulation. BI has been effective in treating coronary diseases but seems to help with most conditions. This inner-vascular system uses a quartz fiber optic cable that gets inserted into a vein through a 10 millimeter needle, and then illuminating a 633nm red laser.

Light therapy has found a prominent position at the State University Medical Center in Georgia, Russia where basic methods of treatment are intravenous laser blood irradiation (ILBI) and non-invasive trans-dermal blood irradiation (TDBI). Studies were conducted to determine the efficacy of non-medicated treatment. In one study, people suffering from poor circulation were treated seven to ten times daily with ILBI. The researchers found normalization in microcirculation disturbances. In another study with pregnant women, the main objective was to avoid adverse side effects of medication and minimize any pharmacological impact on the developing fetus.[159] The study was comprehensive, outlining BI treatment for various indications including:

- vomiting
- disturbances in fetal growth
- labor induction
- chronic urogenital infections
- herpes-virus infection
- toxoplasmotis

It was concluded that BI's "potentialities in the gynecological practice are limitless." It was also found that ILBI therapy averted patients from surgery, required fewer anesthetics and narcotic analgesics following treatment and achieved greater stability and homeostasis (overall health). ILBI also improved blood oxygen levels and normalized heart rhythm. Gastro-intestinal studies were also promising. It was clear that ILBI caused a positive photobiological effect, as there was a corrective influence on pre-cancerous changes in the mucus membrane of the stomach. In cases where patients had cardiovascular and organ infections, IBLI was also effective.

---

[159] Avtandil, Chkheidze, The Evolution of Laser Therapy in Feto-Maternal Medicine, Tbilisi, Georgia.

The reports said the biostimulatory effects of the laser consist of activating the bio-energetic processes of an organism. The Russians reported the following clinical changes:

- increased proliferation activity of human bone marrow cells
- stimulation of DNA
- activated chromosome repair
- fibroblast growth factors (synthesizes collagen, critical in wound healing)
- lymphocyte proliferation (natural killer cells)
- monocytes proliferation (inflammatory responders, immune system)
- granulocytes proliferation (white blood cells)
- blood becomes alkaline, stabilizing pH balance
- resistant neutrophils with enhanced function (first-responders to inflammation)
- stimulation of tissue regeneration
- pathology detoxification effect (ridding of disease)
- thrombolytic action (breaking down of blood clots)
- increased cells' resistance to pathogenic agents (cell stronger against disease)
- stimulation of general and local factors of immune protection
- decreases pathogenicity of microbes and growth of their sensitivity to antibiotics
- normalization of liquid metabolism
- conformational transformation in proteins
- changes in physical and chemical properties of bioliquids
- transportation and membranes properties of organelles and cells
- changes in activity in biochemical reactions

Though discovered years ago, these blood irradiation systems are still in their infancy. Out of all the technologies presented herein, this technology promises to have the greatest impact on the health care systems worldwide.

Both antibiotics and BI were discovered around the same time. It was 1928 when Alexander Fleming came across penicillin in his lab. Antibiotics presented a streamlined approach to medicine; once mass produced, they could be easily transported around the world. Irradiation of a patients' blood, however, had to be conducted with a special device and industrial technology did not have the means or wherewithal for large scale treatments back then. Thus, the use of light in blood irradiation faded into obscurity and did not resurface until recently.

Now, new advances in photobiological technology offer BI the opportunity to take its rightful place in health care. The question is, how long will we have to wait? Perhaps if health care consumers voice their opinions, the medical system will be forced to adapt such innovations.

OPTICAL BRAIN STIMULATION

As if the information presented so far isn't surprising enough, scientists are now using a new technology to interpret the rapid-fire language of the brain with the speed and precision of light. In other words, new light technologies are being used to identify and control brain circuits.

Traditionally, brain function is studied through the use of electrodes. Activating and controlling neuron response with light is much more effective because optogenetics not only maps brain activity, but can control it as well.

Optogenetics allows scientists to study at a single cell level. "From a researcher's standpoint, it is all about selectivity," said Darrin Brager, Ph.D., a research scientist at the University of Texas in Austin. Brager has found optogenetics is brain mapping involving light with more accuracy than ever before. He pointed out that in cases where certain parts of the brain are impaired due to a degenerative condition, there is potential of re-activating or deactivating affected parts of the brain. "In theory, by infusing the light sensitive DNA into areas of interest, then by implanting small chip arrays without damaging the brain, you could activate specific neurons with a pattern of interest or effectiveness."[160] His lab's current focus is figuring out how memory is bio-energetically encoded within the brain and understanding how those processes are altered in diseased states. There is well founded optimism that optogenetic neuroscientists will develop photobiological technologies to treat multiple brain issues such as:

- schizophrenia
- autism

---

[160] Brager D., Interview - Austin, Texas. (2011)

- mental retardation
- epilepsy
- Alzheimer's
- Parkinson's
- depression
- ADHD
- compulsive behaviors
- addiction
- memory loss
- brain trauma

In 2002 neurobiologist Boris Zemelman, Ph.D. began experimenting at the Memorial Sloan-Kettering Cancer Center with light-activated proteins to manipulate neurons. By 2005 at the Department of Cell Biology, Yale University neuroscientist Susana Q. Lima used optogenetics to control a decapitated fly.[161] Optogenetics enables scientists to control behavior by adding or deleting precise activity patterns within animal and insect brains cells. The light can be delivered by using LEDs mounted directly to the skull of the animal or by implanting optical fibers. Optical fibers are effective in delivering light deeper into specific parts of the brain, thus enabling photonic control of neuronal firing.

Zemelman, now part the University of Texas team, is pushing this technology to the next level and theorized an approach to treating drug addiction by locating a particular type of neurotransmitter. Targeting specific types or groups of cells using light as the on/off switch could possibly alleviate the impulse to use drugs. Blue light activates neurons and yellow light quiets them, depending on the proteins used. "Think of it as a universal remote that operates the body's tiniest circuits," commented writer Kara Platoni.[162]

As Associate Professor of Bioengineering and Psychiatry at Stanford, Dr. Karl Deisseroth's interest is investigating the root cause of schizophrenia and other psychotic brain disorders.[163] His associate, Professor Jaimie Henderson focuses on Parkinson's disease, while Professor Krishna Shenoy wants to develop applications to help those with paralysis and

---

[161] Zemelman B., Interview - Austin, Texas. (2011)
[162] Platoni, K. New Light on the Brain. (2010)
[163] Langreth, R. The Light Fantastic. Forbes Magazine (2010)

traumatic head injuries. Stanford is also exploring the brain's sleep-wake neural patterns to understand sleep disorders.

The thought of mind control through electrical stimulation might sound like science fiction, but not for Dr. José Manuel Rodriguez Delgado, formally Physiology Professor at Yale University. His invention, the Stimoceiver, succeeded in using electrical signals to evoke responses in cats, chimpanzees and humans during experiments in the 1960s.[164] He wrote a popular book called *Physical Control of the Mind* in 1969 and was effective in stimulating emotions and controlling behavior with a brain implant. The two-way radio channel system monitored brain waves while sending electrical stimuli. Delgado believes manipulating brain neurons with technology can potentially liberate individuals from psychiatric disorders and innate aggression. His experiments produced a variety of effects including:

- elation
- euphoria
- drowsiness
- alertness
- counteraction of depression
- deep thoughtful concentration
- pleasure
- hilarity
- lust
- fear
- colored visions
- deep relaxation

One of Delgado's patients involuntarily clenched his fist even when he tried to resist. "I guess, Doctor, that your electricity is stronger than my will," he said.[165] Delgado garnered international attention with a demonstration at a bull ranch when he entered the ring with a bull that had been implanted with a Stimoceiver. The animal charged him, but Delgado quickly pressed the remote control to halt the charge, and the bull stopped in its tracks just a few feet away.

---

[164] Delgado, J.M., Permanent Implantation of Multilead Electrodes in the Brain. (1952)
[165] Delgado, J.M., Physical Control of the Mind: Toward a Psychocivilized Society. (1971)

Delgado's research has helped pave the way for modern brain implant technology. Because of the limited drugs available to treat mental illness and recent advances in microchip technology, the resurgence of brain bio-implants is imminent. Delgado asks, "Can you avoid knowledge? You cannot! Things are going ahead in spite of ethics, in spite of your personal beliefs, in spite of everything."[166] In 2010 Stanford University received a 28.8 million dollar DARPA grant to study optogenetics over a four year period. [167] Even DARPA has openly considered implanting brain chips in soldiers to boost their cognitive capabilities.

Lizzie Buchen of *Wired Magazine* wrote an article, "Laser-Controlled Humans Closer to Reality," that opens by stating, "Flashes of light may one day be used to control the human brain, and that day just got a lot closer." Buchen mentions that MIT Lab experiments activated neurons in a monkey's brain, and points out how closely a monkey's brain resembles ours. MIT scientists have also succeeded in exploring and controlling neural circuits in fish, flies, rodents and now in primates.[168]

Buchen states, "Proving the method works in primate brains paves the way not only for better therapies, but also for understanding the relationship between specific neural circuits and behaviors." At Stanford, neuroscientist Edward Boyden pioneered new methods while working with Deisseroth. Boyden makes clear that the use of this technology on primates is safe and causes no damage to the neurons or immune system. Deisseroth points out, "There is a disturbing aspect, too, which raises questions of free will." A video widely circulated among the optogenetics community shows a lab mouse with a fiber optic cable in its head. When the light glows blue, the mouse is compelled to circle left. When the light is turned off, the mouse stops. Is this a remote-controlled mouse?

Botond Roska and her colleagues conducted a successful experiment with blind mice in 2008. The mice responded to light after optogenic treatment.[169] Optical signals were sufficient for the mice to successfully perform optomotor behavioral tasks. In discussing this research

---

[166] Horgan, J., The Myth of Mind Control: Will anyone ever decode the human brain? (2004)
[167] http://landcebu.com/?p=234 Stanford-Led new program aims to produce Insights brain injury, recovery. (2011)
[168] Buchen, L. Laser-Controlled Humans are Closer to Reality. (2009)
[169] Lagali P.S., Balya D., Awatramani G.B., Münch T.A., Kim D.S., Busskamp V., Cepko C.L., Roska B., Light-activated channels targeted to on bipolar cells restore visual function in retinal degeneration. (2008)

experiment Zemelman commented, "It's possible...some types of blindness could be overcome."

According to Zemelman, there are many surprising potential uses for optogenetics. "It's not restricted to the brain. You could cause any organ to do what it does normally, doing it on cue." For example, in diabetes cells are insensitive to sugar, but infusing engineered genetic material into the pancreas and then activating insulin release with light could be promising for diabetics.[170]

Furthermore, Medtronic, the world's largest manufacturer of biomedical technologies, is working toward creating a neural implant approximately the size and shape of a USB flash drive with a wireless data link, a microcontroller, and an optical stimulator. This neural implant uses light to alter the neurons' behavior in the brain.

Cyberkinetics Neurotechnology Systems, Inc. has an FDA-approved "BrainGate" interface that helps disabled patients by sending simple computer commands via direct thoughts designed to move a robotic arm, a computer cursor or even a wheelchair. The hair-thin electrodes sense the electro-magnetic signature of neurons firing in specific areas of the brain.

Another new science, "neural computing," is accomplished by adapting in-vitro cells to a silicon chip, combining sensors and living brain cells. Here, neurons are seeded into a grid of gold electrodes which are connected to a computer. These biochemical engineers from the Universities of Georgia and Florida have been building hybrid robot or 'Hybrot' using neuro-chip technology. Thomas DeMarse and Steven Potter are developing algorithms that harness neuronal responses in situations where living brain cells can be relied upon to make the right decisions. Their goal is to use this technology for un-manned missions, possibly in flight reconnaissance or space.[171]

Utilizing this neuro-chip technology with an optogenetic implant, like a brain inside a brain, could work something like this: cybergenic LED chips with an algorithm pre-programmed to respond to a specific change in a neuron's state, triggering an optogenetic light response which resets the neuron back to a normal state. This "optocybergenetics" system could potentially activate when the brain or organ normal function sputters.

---

[170] Zemelman, B., Interview - Austin, Texas. (2011)
[171] DeMarse, T.B., Wagenaar, D.A., Blau A.W., Potter, S.M, The Neurally Controlled Animat: Biological Brains Acting with Simulated Bodies. (2001)

Watching neurons communicate will help us deduce how brain circuits are laid out. Being able to map neuronal function represents a huge step for health care and science, a prospect that has neuroscientists around the world delving into this new technology. Optogenetics technology has great potential to change the way we view the brain and control neural circuits throughout body.

FUNGAL TREATMENT

Fungal nail infections are estimated to affect more than 35 million Americans. PinPointe USA, Inc., a leader in podiatric light-based therapy, has developed a novel treatment for nail fungus (onychomycosis) using 1064nm wavelength of light. This new photobiological technology is exclusively marketed worldwide by Cynosure, Inc. Nail fungus isn't just a cosmetic problem. For people with diabetes or immune disorders, nail fungus can lead to serious health problems. "With the FDA clearance of the PinPointe FootLaser, patients finally have a pain-free treatment option that is more successful than topically-applied antifungal drugs, safer than oral medication and less painful than surgical removal of the nail," said Dr. Adam Landsman, Assistant Professor of Surgery at Harvard Medical School.

Because the disease lies deep inside the nail, current methods of treatment (topical creams and ointments) in most cases are ineffective. PinPointe's FDA clearance of a proven, patented antimicrobial laser is the first of its type for this indication and boasts a success rate of approximately seventy-five percent. Now, after a single thirty-minute drug-free and painless photobiological treatment, patients can walk out of the office after the session. "Our goal is continued market leadership of podiatric light-based therapeutic technology," said John Strisower, founder and CEO of PinPointe. He worked with leading scientists, medical professionals, and the National Institute of Health for years to develop this technology. Sunlight, as we know, is the original disinfectant, and Strisower's company is seeking to develop light-based disinfectant devices to treat diseases caused by viral, bacteriological and fungal pathogens. Eventually, Strisower hopes to find a treatment for tuberculosis, AIDS and other fatal diseases with photobiological systems.

LASER ACUPUNCTURE

Laser acupuncture is a relatively new method of stimulation that uses low wattage laser beams instead of traditional acupuncture needles to influence the flow of energy at acupuncture points. To be effective, practitioners need a clear understanding of how various acupuncture points function and an in-depth knowledge of traditional Chinese medicine. Laser acupuncture is a bit more esoteric than many of the light treatments discussed previously. There have not been many controlled studies proving that it works, but many practitioners attest to it.

"Laser-puncture" uses lasers instead of needles, alleviating any viral risk in using needles, especially in third world countries where reusing needles is common. There are even user-friendly, intelligent laser puncture systems now available where software automatically recognizes the meridian points and monitors the laser beam for more controlled treatment.

A practitioner typically aims a beam of light onto an acupuncture point to stimulate it, holding the beam steadily for a few seconds to a few minutes, depending on the amount of tissue the laser must penetrate. While deeper abdominal points do not usually benefit from laser puncture, points on a patient's hands, feet, ears and other parts of the body often respond well.

Initial clinical results suggest that laser acupuncture treatments might be more effective than the classical needle approach in some cases. Some practitioners are using this approach as a means to tone the body and bring it up to a higher functioning level in what is called "body energy balancing." Applying a continual light to meridians, acupressure and chakra points, and manually rotating the light-generating device is said to provide results. Monochromatic light applied to the acupuncture points travels through the meridians of the body like fiber optic cables to reach internal areas and organs. In fact, using laser puncture on the bellybutton is purported to improve circulation.

Russian Olympic team psychologist Dr. Gregory Raiport from the National Research Institute of Physical Culture in Moscow is practicing laser-puncture to treat depression, anxiety and addictions. This procedure is also said to be effective in treating painful conditions such as carpal tunnel syndrome, tennis elbow, arthritis, chronic headaches in children and numerous others.

The Russians are also testing laser acupuncture on pregnant woman, again to avoid treatment with drugs or surgery. Several effective photobiological treatments have been found for various complications. Anemia, which can cause miscarriage and immature delivery, has a treatment length of between three to ten days, with a light exposure of 10 to 30 seconds at each point. In cases of arterial hypotonia (abnormally low blood pressure), the exposure was 30 to 40 seconds at each point, three to seven times over a week. In situations when ovarian hypofunction threatened miscarriage, women were treated with light in order to stimulate endogenic hormone production. The exposure time on each point was 10 to 15 seconds with eight to eleven treatments.

Laser acupuncture is also effective for smoking cessation treatments and can reduce cravings for nicotine, ease withdrawal symptoms and stimulate the body's ability to detoxify from nicotine. The FDA, however, considers laser therapy for quitting smoking experimental, due to the lack of properly documented research, even though there are no side effects and many patients report positive results.

It is important to note that a major benefit of light-based technologies is the lack of toxic side effects. Another benefit is that light treatment is inexpensive. Once the equipment is paid for, the operation cost is minimal. It's just a matter of time before these affordable and effective systems of treatment will become available. Luckily, these new technologies are backed by experts ranging from people at the FDA to the American Cancer Society; the health care system now must embrace them. The question is what will it take to get there?

Chapter Four: Cosmetic Light Treatments

Everyone wants to look younger, and this desire has fueled an immense growth in the cosmetics industry. Light treatments show promising results in cosmetic procedures. United States dermatologists currently perform an estimated 60 million anti-aging treatments a year, and this trend is growing. According to Linda Boyd, in an article found in Duke University's archives, the cosmetics industry "totals over 20 billion in sales."[172] Traditional creams, facial peels, surgeries, chemical injections and drugs are typically expensive and can also be dangerous, often causing scarring, nerve problems and possibly death, due to many factors including surgery, astringent chemicals and compounds that are out of sync with our bodies' natural processes.

Educated consumers want natural, noninvasive methods to satisfy their cosmetic needs, and light treatments provide a solution. Light offers new alternatives that cosmetic companies are just now beginning to seriously address. In some cases, light technologies create visible photobiological improvements that can be noticed after a few treatments.

CHEMICALS IN COSMETICS

Biomonitoring tests can find hundreds of manmade chemicals in the body.[173] Some of these toxins are known carcinogens. The big mystery is how did these chemicals get there?[174] The cosmetics industry has been hammered from every direction by individuals, consumer groups and legislators and currently there is still little FDA oversight. Stacy Malkan's book *Not Just a Pretty Face* unveils an industry that operates in secrecy. In the United States cosmetic manufactures are free to compound chemicals and market them without FDA approval.

Several countries including Japan, China and Europe restrict the use of many toxic chemicals. There is a clear link from many of the toxic chemicals used in skin, hair and cosmetics products, to cancer, birth defects

---

[172] http://library.duke.edu/digitalcollections/adaccess/guide/cosmetics
[173] Centers for Disease Control and Prevention. "Natural Report on Human Exposure to Environmental Chemicals." www.cdc.gov/exposurereport Also - Environmental Working Group. "Human Taxome Project: Mapping the Pollution in People. www. bodyburden.org.
[174] Fischer, Douglas, "What's in You?" Oakland Tribune. (2006)

and learning disabilities.[175] In 1999 the European Union (E.U.) banned the use of specific carcinogenic and hormonal disruptive chemicals in cosmetic products.[176] Activists in the United States attempted to pass similar legislation but did not succeed due to the huge cosmetics industry lobby.

One of the first leaders in green chemistry, Amy Cannon, Ph. D. developed a great replacement for toxic hair straightening products. One of her innovations uses UV light to shrink wrap hair into a non-toxic perm. This system is known as "water-soluble photocrosslinking materials in cosmetics." It won an award for best paper at the 2006 Society of Cosmetic Chemists.[177] She has been credited as coming up with one of the most innovative ideas in "green" cosmetic chemistry. When discussing hair perms, Cannon said, "It's some of the most toxic chemistry out there…never mind putting it on your hair." Hopefully with public awareness, ideas like these will take hold in the market and spur new innovations that do not have potentially adverse effects on health.

ANTI-AGING

Light Emitting Diodes or low wattage lasers can penetrate deep below the surface of the skin without causing damage. This method of photobiological treatment encourages the rejuvenation of dermal tissue. In a 2002 article, "Balance You Hormones and Erase Wrinkles" in *Woman's World Magazine*, David Olszewski writes, "Just one hour of red light treatment daily stimulates the formation of new skin cells and skin-firming collagen; improvements can be seen in just 24 hours." Light therapy is a powerful anti-aging tool. As we age we begin to see effects like wrinkles, enlarged pores, crow's feet and age spots. This is due in part to decreased collagen levels in the skin accelerated by the process of aging and lifestyle factors such as smoking, tanning, stress management and diet.

Light activates the chemical energy ATP (adenosine triphosphate) within cells and also activates collagen and elastin production. Collagen is then pulled towards the skin's surface as it proliferates, rises and fills in the wrinkles. Heeral R. Shah, M.D. and Michael T. Yen, M.D. of the Baylor

---

[175] Malkan, Stacy, "Not Just A Pretty Face" New Society Publishers. (2007)
[176] www.ec.europa.eu/consumers/safety/prod_legis/index_en.htm
www.leffingwell.com/cosmetics/vol_1en.pdf
[177] The Society of Cosmetic Chemist won the best an award for best paper to Amy Cannon, Ph.D.
"Water-Soluble Photocrosslinking Materials in Cosmetics" at the Annual Scientific Seminar. (2006)

College of Medicine firmly believe that, "the non-thermal light treatment stimulates fibroblast proliferation, collagen synthesis and growth factors."

Light therapy biostimulation helps improve damaged skin and makes it firmer and tighter. It is found that low-powered lasers and LEDs improve blemishes and give the skin greater elasticity and texture for a healthier, youthful appearance.

DO-IT-YOURSELF TREATMENTS

Light could play a significant role in new photobiological treatments without the assistance of a dermatologist. L'Oreal, Avon, Proctor & Gamble and Johnson & Johnson are seeing this new trend in do-it-yourself dermatology.[178] Soon people will be able to remove age spots, acne, and wrinkles without the assistance of a medical professional.

Currently cosmetic companies are marketing their products as part of a virtual at-home or do-it-yourself salon. At-home hair removal and acne devices are already on the shelves. Palomar Medical Technology jumped into a $120 million deal with Johnson & Johnson's Neutrogena Brand to develop a handheld light-based device that treats wrinkles, cellulite and acne, although to my knowledge, it was never released.

Palomar's C.F.O. Paul Weiner believes they are in position to penetrate a good part of the market. Proctor & Gamble also worked with Israeli medical device manufacturer, Syneron Medical, Ltd., to develop devices that use radio frequency and light to combat the signs of aging, another do-it-yourself treatment.

Ageless Beauty President and C.E.O. Maha Sherifis is marketing light devices in several wavelengths with specific dermal indications: blue to treat acne, green anti-inflammatory to promote healing, red to encourage collagen production, infrared to even out skin tone and reduce redness and age spots.

Pharos Life Founder and C.E.O. John Kennedy markets a handheld home-use light therapy device called Tända. His handheld unit has interchangeable heads in three different wavelength of light at blue, red, and

---

[178] www.time.com/time/magazine/article/0,9171,1666284,00.html

infrared. Pharos has also developed pre-treatment topical gels to reduce reflection and facilitate optimal delivery of the light.

L'Oreal is the largest beauty and cosmetics company in the world. They collaborated with Light BioScience, LLC to develop Photomodulation® devices for skincare using Light BioScience proprietary skin rejuvenation technology to reduce wrinkles and the visible signs of aging. "We have decided to pool our in-depth knowledge of skin and Light BioScience's unique expertise in Photomodulation® to offer consumers a new and complementary approach to skincare," says Jean-François Grollier, L'Oreal's executive vice president research and development.[179] This project spawned the opening of a new research and development division at L'Oreal. "We are very excited about this agreement. We can take advantage of the support of the world's leading cosmetics research force to jointly develop some new and highly promising applications in skin devices," says Rick Krupnick, CEO at Light BioScience.

Krucpnick also pointed out their GentleWaves® is the first FDA-approved LED device to effectively treat periorbital (around the eyes) wrinkles.[180] According to Dr. McDaniel, the senior developer on the project and Director of the Institute of Anti-Aging Research in Virginia Beach, Virginia, the unit has a pulse setting, and treatments can take anywhere from thirty-five seconds to a few minutes. It operates in both yellow and infrared wavelengths. The treatment protocol is a couple of sessions per week with a total of eight to twelve required. The GentleWaves® device is designed for salon application, but there was a mention of a home-based unit. "Patients have been waiting for a gentle, pain-free skin fitness regime without side effects, downtime or a huge investment," says Krucpnick.

Robert A. Weiss, M.D., Associate Professor of Dermatology at Johns Hopkins University School of Medicine said, "For the first time, we are both slowing down collagen breakdown and building up new collagen with no pain, no redness, and no serious side effects GentleWaves® unique ability to stimulate and/or inhibit cell signaling pathways for skin rejuvenation truly represents the next frontier in anti-aging medicine." Here once again, to my knowledge, this new photobiological light therapy device was never released and the GentleWaves® system has been taken off the market. What is the hold up in getting these devices out to market?

---

[179] www.ia-ar.com/press/press_release_light_bioscience_final.pdf
[180] www.news-medical.net/news/2005/01/05/7135.aspx

HYPER-PIGMENTATION AND DERMAL ISSUES

In most cases hyper-pigmentation is associated with the aging process. Now there is new photobiological technology to treat this issue. Using photons of light energy can normalize the melanin that causes dark spots. This form of light therapy can be effective in minimizing sun spots, acne scars, large pores and other visible spot irregularities. In an article from Livestrong.com, Dr. Harvey Jay points out that pulsed light therapy can be used to treat skin discolorations ranging from dark to light and areas where collected pigment has caused raised, thickened skin. "Pulsed light lasers are successful in treating brown spots, port wine stains (skin discoloration) and areas of redness due to sun damage." [181]

Physicians have been using light for stretch marks, burns and scars with great results. Solta Medical Inc. developed the Fraxel Dual® laser, a combination of 1550nm and 1927nm laser light that reaches deep into the dermis to stimulate collagen remodeling by removing top layers of the skin, usually several grams during a session. The addition of both wavelengths in a single treatment makes the improvements faster and increases its effectiveness. A full-face treatment is typically completed in less than an hour, and results can be clearly seen a few weeks after treatment. After the scabbing heals, patients generally look as if they have lost years off their faces. Most of the effect on the dermis occurs as a result of the hot laser mechanism that removes the surface layer of the skin, but it is considered a non-ablative treatment.

"Complementing the Fraxel Dual with post dermal biostimulation light therapy sessions could accelerate client recovery time significantly," said Devon Perry L.M.E. who owns My Skincare Boutique in Austin, Texas. There are a handful of aesthetic laser devices available for this type of skin treatment, but Solta Medical released the first dual laser system on the market.

The Fraxel device has also been approved to treat Actinic Keratosis (AK), which are considered pre-cancerous skin cells, also known as skin tags. A six-month clinical study of twenty-one subjects found there was an 83.5 percent reduction of AK lesions using the dual laser. These treatments were effective on the face, arms, hands and chest area. Subjects underwent a series of two to four treatments over an average of three weeks without adverse reaction. "In our study, we found the Fraxel to be the most effective treatment of multiple facial AKs, as it is safe and requires minimal downtime while simultaneously improving other signs of photodamage," said Roy G. Geronemus, M. D. and Director of the Laser & Skin Surgery Center of New York. "While the removal rate was comparable to other topical therapies and AK treatment options, Fraxel was overwhelmingly well-tolerated by all the patients and offers the added benefit of improving a patients' overall skin quality, color and texture. My patients will now have an effective and safe treatment option for the removal of precancerous lesions on their face as well as on the body," said Suzanne L. Kilmer, M.D. and founder of the Laser & Skin Surgery Center of Northern California. Stephen J. Fanning, CEO of Solta Medical, Inc. asserts, "We are providing our physicians with cutting-edge technology that patients are seeking, specifically in terms of reversing sun damage and treating precancerous skin lesions."

VASCULAR LESIONS

Light also treats vascular lesions such as spider, varicose and threat veins by increasing circulation and the formation of new capillaries needed to replace the damaged ones. The treatment targets a specific hemoglobin pigment in the blood, normalizing the cells and eliminating their unsightly appearance from the skin, once again without causing damage to the epidermis.

A photobiological device in the Biolitec AG arsenal is the ELVeS® (Endo Laser Vein System). This is possibly the most effective way to treat varicose veins on the market. There is no postoperative pain, swelling, or bruising, as well as no recovery period. The probe is inserted through a small entry into the vein to be treated. It then photothermically seals the varicose expanded vein. It is the world's first radial (360°) emitting laser fiber, producing excellent clinical cosmetic results with minimum discomfort.

ACNE TREATMENT

Light systems specifically designed to treat acne typically utilize blue light, which has been found highly effective. The epidermis absorbs the light, which triggers a response and destroys the acne-causing bacteria. Following the session with red light is also effective in reducing dermal inflammation associated with acne and also speeds up the healing process. In combination, both red and blue light can be highly effective tools in combating acne. In the early 2000's the FDA began approving these devices which are currently available from several manufacturers.

CELLULITE AND WEIGHT REDUCTION

Most people would give anything to get rid of cellulite. Cellulite is caused by a number of factors, including genetics, age, pregnancy, eating habits and metabolic disorders. Cellulite is difficult to shed because it has formed around muscle and bone. Light therapy aids in the diminishing of cellulite by improving microcirculation of lymph nodes and blood flow.

Veronica Stetson, a massage therapist in Scottsdale, Arizona uses an LED light therapy device on cellulite. In an article "The Light Fantastic for Day Spa" for *DaySpa Magazine*, Stetson states that she usually has to use an aggressive deep tissue massage technique which is often painful for clients, especially if they suffer from "hard" cellulite. After the spa acquired a light therapy device to treat clients with cellulite problems, Stetson noticed she only had to give a superficial massage when also employing light therapy. The results are significantly better, Stetson states, and there is less swelling in the lymph nodes and better circulation.

Furthermore, Kim Segal, another innovator in light therapy, has been using cold laser treatments to help patients lose weight. Light therapy with cold laser treatments releases endorphins, which helps to suppress appetite and reduce cravings. The endorphin rush also boosts metabolism and mitigates the depression and stress that often come with dieting.

HAIR REGENERATION

People who struggle with premature hair loss truly benefit from light therapy. While high wattage lasers are used for hair removal, low wattage lasers or LEDs can be used to promote hair growth. In 2007, the FDA cleared the first hand-held laser therapy device designed to treat hair loss. The light treatment allows for photon energy to activate enzymes found within the body that normalize damaged tissue. Improved blood flow leads to an increase in the number of corpuscles that give oxygen and nutrients to a damaged hair root bulb. The photobiological result is production of stronger, healthier and faster-growing hair shafts as well as a healthier scalp.

Light can also regenerate hair follicles damaged from waxing or tweezing, facilitate growth, and undo uneven or otherwise bad hair removal work.

Laser combs also promote hair growth. Each unit contains several panels of lasers, akin to comb teeth, that shine light onto the scalp. In this noninvasive treatment, the therapeutic light is absorbed by the cells in the scalp and the process of cell repair begins. European studies of this procedure have shown that in fifty-five percent of these cases, light therapy actually stimulates new hair growth. There are a number of laser combs on the market; one is the HairMax Laser Comb that has nine beams that send light into the scalp to improve hair condition and energize hair follicles. In 2000, the HairMax device was named one of the inventions of the year by *Time Magazine.*

Light therapy offers a safer, more affordable alternative to traditional and invasive treatments. If you take a closer look at the benefits, it becomes evident why light therapies are getting serious attention. The use of light appears to be the future of cosmetics, and any entrepreneurs recognizing this could reap the benefits. Light treatment enhances epidermal tissue, working with the body's natural processes to rejuvenate it to an optimum state. Light works with the cells' natural processes and is generally safe for all skin types. The cosmetic industry is slowly recognizing that using environmentally friendly products is better for consumers and the planet. With consumer-awareness at an all-time high, people are now seeing that chemicals, invasive surgery and ablative therapy are outdated and in some cases dangerous treatments. Light offers a safer, affordable and effective alternative.

CONCLUSION

The quest to understand and develop uses for light, most likely, will never end. I believe the deeper we probe into the mysteries surrounding light, the more sophisticated light applications will become. Harnessing light technology will soon become an important commodity in health care around the world, leading us to find cures for ailments and disease that we never thought possible.

Throughout history our connection to light has been a constant source of health and empowerment. Modern science allows for a deeper understanding of light's properties, and we have taken that information to find various ways to utilize its energy for practical purposes. Now, to discover that all living cells emanate light as a part of a vast, complex communication network, is nothing short of amazing. The exciting discoveries made in just the past century promise groundbreaking results in studies to come.

For example, we are now beginning to view the sun and its radiant energy differently with all of the new information being published. There is certainly no denying sunlight's importance to our health. Vitamin D is crucial for healthy functioning and the best way to obtain the amount of vitamin D our bodies need is from pure, unblocked sunlight, the way nature intended, and not from manufactured supplements.

Likewise, to think that artificial light (non-full spectrum light) could have such an adverse effect on human health is a bit dumbfounding, if not disturbing. Non-full spectrum artificial light has a negative impact on our endocrine systems and could possibly lead to such ailments as seasonal affective disorder, depression, eyestrain headaches and cancer in susceptible individuals. Clearly, with so many people working indoors under artificial light conditions, more research needs to be conducted and steps taken to rectify this potential health hazard.

Ultraviolet (UV) light has many applications as well, ranging from treating jaundiced babies to purifying water and air. If the studies on blood irradiation prove accurate, health care systems around the world could save billions of dollars. Using this technology would undoubtedly disrupt the status quo of the industrial pharmaceutical complex. To dream even bigger, it is possible sunlight's UV rays could be used to eliminate blood-borne pathogens in third-world countries, thus reducing the need for expensive UV blood eradiation medical equipment.

Clearly light technologies have the potential to revolutionize medicine. My hope is that this book will educate people about new available medical treatment options, and act as a catalyst for new ideas inspiring innovative development. Integrating this technology into the mainstream medical community is the next step. Other countries are already harnessing light technologies; now the United States needs to realize the health and economic benefits these technologies make possible.

The traditional medical model practiced in the United States profits from illness, rather than wellness. The reason is simple: There is money to be made from illness. Profiting from people's illnesses, however, presents several issues and the pitfalls outweigh the benefits. According to the World Health Organization, the United States currently ranks 37th in the world for health care, it can do better than this.

The American medical system is heavily influenced by politics, economics, insurance companies and the pharmaceutical industry. The fact that many FDA regulators who are paid to protect Americans' rights have worked for the very companies they are supposed to regulate, and in many cases, are later rehired by these same companies. The conflicts of interest are clear. Universities taking contributions from pharmaceutical companies for research (peer-reviewed studies) will also feel the pressures of bias. Politicians making legislative and appointment decisions will subjugate to special interest groups that help fund their campaigns.

The American health care system is sick. One idea I have come up with to cut out the bureaucracy, doctor gouging and drug exploitation is for large hospitals to offer their own insurance. While this is not an original idea, I believe it will help. The only hospital system in the world using this business model is Kaiser Permanente which has become the biggest managed care consortium in the world. From its inception, Kaiser Permanente strongly supports preventive medicine dedicating itself in the education of its members about maintaining their own health.

Fortune magazine had reported in 1944 that 90% of the U.S. citizens could not afford 'fee-for-service' healthcare. (Sound familiar?) After World War II Kaiser health care was offered to the public and became a great success. However, the American Medical Association (AMA) opposed the Kaiser system of managed care from the very beginning and attempted to defuse demand for Kaiser Permanente managed care by promoting the expansion of the Blue Cross and Blue Shield. Kaiser fought off AMA attacks and eventually triumphed. Kaiser was not the first to have come nose-to-nose with the AMA; Presidents Roosevelt and Truman also faced strong opposition when trying to implement medical programs to benefit the American public.

Kaiser Permanente's success has been attributed to three practices:

- A strong emphasis on preventive care, reducing costs later on (in their best interest because they are the insurance holder).
- Doctors are salaried rather than paid per service, which removes the incentive for doctors to perform unnecessary procedures and surgeries.
- Minimizing the time patients spend in costly hospitals by careful planning and shifting care to outpatient clinics.

These practices save Kaiser Permanente money enabling lower costs for patients and its members. Kaiser Permanente realized early on keeping people healthy saves money and requires less hospitalization. Studies have shown Kaiser patients spend on average less time in their hospitals. A 2004 *New York Times* article, "Is Kaiser the Future of American Health Care?"[182] points outs that medical doctors are fed up with the bureaucracy of the current medical system, and how Kaiser Permanente manages their patients' health, not just their illnesses.

There are doctors throughout the world who really want to heal people, but they are part of a system in which their hands are tied. It is time for a change, and there are many new technologies for restoring health. Now more than ever, there is an urgency to address integrative, complementary, alternative and naturopathic types of medicine.

The United States National Institute of Health (NIH) made a failed attempt in 1991 to launch the National Center for Complementary and Alternative Medical. It was disappointing because of the positive expectations for this organization. But bureaucrats stood in the way. The powers that be did not want the organization to succeed. Naturopathic methods such as light, vitamins, herbs, amino acids, nutrient therapies are a threat to the pharmaceutical industry because they cannot be patented and this translates into potential profit loss.

It is time for humanity to take responsibility for our personal health. We need to become proactive. Write your legislative representatives, create a blog advocating what you believe in, volunteer with a local health advocacy organization or start one, coordinate local CAM group, promote lectures, pressure local media to produce and publish more stories on CAM. Or face the alternative: living within a broken medical system.

Each one of us can make a difference; small steps can make big impacts. Educating people about this information will drive these new photobiological technologies into the market, making them available and affordable. We cannot allow these innovations to sit in the shadows. Currently, there are a handful of practitioners, doctors, university scientists and government regulators who know how effective technologies are.

Light is the basis of all life. From the earliest one cell incarnations, light has played a pivotal role in our evolution. It has been a major influence

---

[182] Lohr, Steve, "Is Kaiser the Future of America Health Care" (October 2004)

every step of the way, so it makes sense it would play such an important part in the regulation, communication and healing of our bodies.

These new systems of medical treatment have the potential to help the ailing health care system potentially making health care affordable for everyone. Just think, medical treatment having the ability to reduce or eliminate drug intake, less drugs in many cases equates to lower health care costs. Many of the light treatments can be done for pennies on the dollar. This also saves people from the counter indicated side effects of drug use, which can eventually equate to additional future costs and health issues. These technologies also reduce the need for invasive surgeries in many cases and can reduce the incidence of infections. Light-based healing technologies will become more affordable and eventually find their way into every hospital, ambulance and emergency room. Then, eventually into people's homes, thus averting doctor and hospital visits, reducing health care expenses, keeping people healthier, wealthier and happier.

Glossary

Actinin Keratosis: Also know as skin tags are considered a pre-cancerous condition with a twenty percent risk of becoming malignant.

Aeruginosa: A common bacterium found in soil, water and skin flora and thriving on most surfaces causing disease in all animals, including humans.

Aesthetic: Sensory or sensori-emotional values study.

Alkalinity: Measure of the ability of a solution to neutralize acid.

Aminolevulinic Acid (ALA): is the first compound in porphyrins (group of organic compounds of which many occur in nature) synthesis pathway leading to heme in mammals and chlorophyll in plants.

Amotosalen: A light-activated, DNA and RNA-crosslinking psoralen compound, which is used to neutralize pathogens.

Analgesics: Any drugs used to relieve pain.

Antibiotic-resistance genes: The genes offering to bacteria and other microorganisms the possibility of resisting an antibiotic to which they were once sensitive.

Antibodies: A protein used by the immune system to identify and neutralize foreign objects such as bacteria and viruses.

Antimicrobial: A substance that kills or prevents the growth of microorganisms.

Arterial plaque: A fatty deposit inside an arterial wall.

Arteriosclerosis (hardening of the arties): Refers to any hardening and loss of elasticity of medium or large arteries.

ATP (adenosine triphosphate): Transforms energy within cells. A high-energy phosphate molecule constituting the source of energy for your body.

Atraumatic: Not causing trauma or damage.

Bacteria: Single-celled microorganisms which can exist either independently or as parasites.

Bilirubin: A yellow-orange compound produced by the breakdown of hemoglobin from red blood cells.

Biochemical: The process applying tools and concepts of chemistry to living systems.

Biodefenses: The use of biological agents to take defensive measures against attacks.

Bioenergic Processes: Processes involved in making and breaking of chemical bonds in the molecules found in biological organisms with the energy.

Biological Agents: Any bacterium or virus or toxin that could be used in biological warfare.

Bioluminescence: The process by which any living organism produces or emits light.

Biophoton: A photon of light emitted by all biological systems.

Biostimulation: Involves exposing living tissues to specific waves of light creating a photobiological reaction that accelerates cellular homeostasis.

Biosurveillance: Is a set of methods used to detect and measure the concentration of pollutants or their metabolites within the different levels of biological organization.

Bioterrorism: Use of biological agents to lead terrorist attacks.

Biowar: Causing death or injury to humans, animals, or plants by using of disease-producing microorganisms, toxic biological products, or organic biocides.

Botulism: A severe, sometimes fatal food poisoning caused by ingestion of food containing botulin.

Bronchoscope: An instrument for examining and providing access to the interior of the bronchial tubes.

Caged Neurotransmitters: Molecules that are transformed to a neuroactive state by exposure to light of an appropriate wavelength and intensity in order to send nerve signals across a synapse between two neurons.

Calcitriol: The physiologically active form of vitamin D formed primarily in the kidney.

Candela: International system of unit used to measure luminous intensity.

Capillaries: Refer to the smallest of a body's blood vessels connecting arterioles and venules and enable the exchange many important nutrient and waste chemical substances between blood and surrounding tissues.

Chemiluminescence: A chemical reaction leading to emitting light with limited emission of heat.

Chemotherapy: The chemical treatment of an ailment by killing micro-organisms or cancerous cells.

Chlorophyll: Any of a group of green pigments that are found in the chloroplasts of plants and in other photosynthetic organisms.

Cholecalciferol: A form of vitamin D.

Chronobiological: A study that examines periodic and cyclic phenomena in living organisms and their adaptation to solar and lunar related rhythms.

Circadian: Refers to events occurring within a 24-hour period, in the span of a full day, and is a fundamental property possessed by all organisms.

Coherence: The correlation of waves/a wave in phase (unison) without or minimal interference.

Collagen: A group of naturally occurring proteins that constitutes the main component of connective tissue.

Corticosteroid: Are a class of steroid hormones involved in a wide range of physiologic systems such as stress response, immune response and regulation of inflammation.

Cosmeceutical: Refers to the marriage of cosmetics and pharmaceuticals.

Cuvette: Small tube of circular or square cross section, sealed at one end, made of plastic, glass, or fused quartz used for UV light and designed to hold samples for spectroscopic experiments.

Cytochromes: Membrane-bound hemoproteins that contain heme groups and carry out electron transport.

Dihydroxyvitamin: A compound physiologically active as metabolite of vitamin D to regulate calcium metabolism, alkaline phosphatase activity, and enhances the calcemic effect of calcitril.

Dysplasia: A term used in pathology to refer to an abnormal growth in cells development.

Elastin: An elastic protein found in connective tissue that allows body tissues to resume their shape after stretching or contracting.

Electrodes: Electrical conductors used to make contact with a nonmetallic part of a circuit.

Electrodynamics: The study of moving electric charges and their interaction with magnetic and electric fields.

Electromagnetic Radiation: A form of energy that shows wave-like behavior as it travels through space.

Electromagnetic Spectrum: The range of all possible frequencies of electromagnetic radiation.

Electrophysiology: The study of the electrical properties of biological cells and tissues.

Electrostimulation: Shocks of electricity administered in no convulsive doses.

Endocrine System: The glands' information signal system using hormones to assure communication between cells.

Endorphins: A morphine-like substance originating from within the body during exercise, excitement, pain, consumption of spicy food, love and orgasm to produce analgesia and a feeling of well-being.

Endovaginal: High-resolution probe that retrieves images of the uterus and ovaries.

Enzymes: Are proteins that increase the rates chemical reactions.

Erysipelas: A bacterial infection of the skin and subcutaneous tissue, usually involving the face, ears and lower legs.

Exfoliating: A chemical or mechanical process involving the removal of the oldest dead skin cells on the skin's outermost surface.

Exophthalmus: A unilateral or bilateral bulging of the eye interiorly out of the eye orbit.

Extracorporeal: Refers to outside the body in the anatomic sense.

Extracorporeal Photo-Phoresis: An immune-modulatory therapy that is used for the treatment of diseases such as cutaneous T-cell lymphoma.

Feces: Is a waste product from an animal's digestive tract expelled through the anus during defecation.

Fibroblastic Activity: Activity linked to fibroblast which is a cell found within fibrous connective tissues associated with the formation of collagen fibers and ground substance of connective tissue.

Fibroblasts: Cell found within fibrous connective tissues associated with the formation of collagen fibers and ground substance of connective tissue.

Free Radical: Any atom or molecule that has a single unpaired electron in an outer shell. The free-radical theory of aging states that organisms age because cells accumulate free radical damage over time.

Garrulousness: Excessively talking about unimportant things.

Glutamate: A receptor on the membrane of cells, building block of proteins.

Granulocytes: a category of the white blood cells filled with microscopic granules containing enzymes, compounds that digest microorganisms.

Helium-Neon: A common gas used in old lasers.

Hematology: Branch of internal medicine concerned with the study of blood.

Hematoporphyrin: Iron-free derivative of heme obtained by treating hemoglobin with sulfuric acid in vitro and used as an antidepressant and antipsychotic.

Hemoglobin: The oxygen-carrying pigment of red blood cells that gives them their red color and serves to convey oxygen to the tissues.

Hertz (Hz): International system unit of frequency of one cycle per second for a periodic phenomenon.

Homeostasis: A healthy cell or group of cells, maintaining a system of balance, operating within a normal range of function.

Hyperbilirubinemia: An elevated level of the pigment bilirubin in the blood which can lead to death.

Hyper-Pigmentation: The darkening of an area of skin or nails caused by increased melanin due to sun damage, inflammation, or other skin injuries.

Hypertension: Elevation of the systemic arterial blood pressure.

Hypothalamus: A portion of the brain that links the nervous system to the endocrine system among other things.

Immune Modulation: A field in the medical treatment of viral infections applied by introducing an agent into the body that boosts specific areas of the immune system.

Immune Response: Refers to how the body detects foreign and harmful substances to defend against bacteria and viruses.

Immunostimulants: Substances – whether drugs or nutrients that stimulate the immune system by inducing activation or increasing activity of any of its components.

Infrared Light: Is part of the electromagnetic wave spectrum that borders the lowest frequency/longest wavelength among those that make up visible light.

Intravenously: Administration of substances into vein.

In Vitro: An organism that have been isolated from its natural biological environment for experimentation.

Invasive: Tending to intrude, to penetrate healthy tissue by entry with needle.

Irradiating: Process by which treatment or effect is made by application of radiation energy.

IU (international unit): An amount of substance based on biological activity, a relative measure.

Joule (metric SI): Unit of energy expended at one meter per second.

Kelvin Rating: Referring to Kelvin which is the unit used to measure the temperature. The rating is associated to the color of light emitted.

Kinetic: The energy a object possesses relative to its motion.

Lactic Acid: A chemical compound that plays a role in several biochemical processes.

Light Therapy: Body exposure therapy to daylight or specific wavelengths of light for healing purposes.

Light-Active Chemicals: Use of light to activate the energy necessary for a chemical reaction.

Liposome: An artificial microscopic vesicle used to convey vaccines, drugs, enzymes, or other substances to target cells or organs.

Lumens: Measurement unit for the power of light as perceived by the human eye.

Luminous Flux: A quantitative expression to the brilliance of different wavelengths visible light as seen by the human eye.

Lux: Measurement unit of luminance and luminous intensity, watts per square meter.

Lymphatic system: Part of the immune system, it consists of organs, ducts, and nodes to transports a watery clear to distribute immune cells and other factors throughout the body.

Lymphocytes: A small white blood cell that plays a large role in defending the body against disease.

Macular Degeneration: A medical condition that results in a loss of vision in the center of the visual field because of damage to the retina.

Malignant: The tendency of a medical condition to become progressively worse and to potentially result in death.

Mal-Illuminated: Not well exposed to solar radiation or full spectrum light.

Melatonin: A hormone produced by the pineal gland that plays a role in sleep, aging, and reproduction in mammals.

Metabolism: Processing of substances within the living body.

Methoxypsoralen: A compound naturally found in several species of plants. It is a photoactive substance that forms DNA adducts in the presence of ultraviolet radiation.

Microbes: A microorganism, can be a health or pathogenic bacterium.

Microbiology: The study of microorganisms, which are microscopic, unicellular, and cell-cluster organisms. It usually includes the study of the immune system.

Microdermabrasion : A non-invasive method for facial rejuvenation that removes away the outermost layer of dead skin cells from the epidermis.

Mitochondria: Structures responsible for energy production in cells.

Molecule: The smallest particle of a substance that retains the chemical and physical properties of the substance.

Monochromatic: A single wavelength of light radiation.

Monocyte: A type of white blood cell constituting among other things the human body's immune system.

Monotheism: Basing belief that only one god exists.

Morphogenetic field: A group of cells able to respond to discrete, localized biochemical signals leading to the development of specific morphological structures or organs.

Mutations: Changes in an organism's hereditary information.

Nanometer: A measurement unit for light and length of wave used for very small lengths and equal to one billionth of a meter.

Necrotizing: Causing the death of a specific area of tissue.

Neurobiology: The biological study of the nervous system.

Neurodegenerative: A loss of structure and function or death of neurons.

Neurology: A medical specialty dealing with disorders of the nervous system.

Neuromodulation: Electrical stimulation of a peripheral nerve, the spinal cord, or the brain for relief of pain.

Neurons: An electrically excitable cell that processes and transmits information by electrical and chemical signaling.

Neuroscience: Scientific study of the nervous system.

Neutrophil: A type of white blood cell that helps the cell to kill and digest microorganisms it has engulfed.

Nitric Oxide: A chemical gas considered as an important cell signaling molecule in mammals.

Nits: A measure for the luminance unit. It is to 1 candle per square meter measured perpendicular to the rays from the source.

Optical Biopsy: A technique that uses the interaction of light and tissue to provide information about cells.

Optogenetics: A field combining optical and genetic techniques to probe neural circuits within intact mammals and other animals to understand neural information processing.

Optomotor Response: An innate behavior common to all insects that serves for course stabilization during free locomotion. The purpose of this behavior is to regain the desired course of locomotion.

Organelles: A specialized subunit within a cell that has a specific function.

Organism: An individual living thing that can react to stimuli, reproduce and grow. It can be a virus, bacterium, fungus, plant or an animal.

Osteomalacia: The softening of the bones due to defective bone mineralization secondary to inadequate amounts of available phosphorus and calcium.

Oxidation: The combination of a substance with oxygen that creates a reaction in which the atoms in an element lose electrons and the valence of the element are correspondingly increased.

pH: (balance) Measure of aqueous solutions in order balance acidity and basicity.

Pandemic: An epidemic of infectious disease that is spreading through human populations across a large region.

Pathogenicity: The ability of a pathogen to produce an infectious disease in an organism.

Pathogen: A biological agent such as a virus, bacteria or fungus that causes disease to its host.

Pathology: The study and diagnosis of disease.

Periodontal Disease: Diseases that effect one or more of the tissues that both surround and support the teeth.

Periorbital: Area situated around the eye.

Petri Dish: A shallow glass or plastic cylindrical lidded dish used to culture cells or small moss plants.

Phagocytes: the white blood cells that protect the body by ingesting harmful foreign particles, bacteria, and dead or dying cells.

Pheresing: A process wherein blood in drawn and separated.

Photobiological: The biological response light has on cells that result in chemical or physical changes. A term commonly used in the description of light therapy treatments.

Phosphene: Flashes of light induced by movement or sound; the phenomenon is characterized by the experience of seeing light without light actually entering the eye.

Photobiology: The scientific study of the interactions of light and living organisms.

Photochemistry: The study that describes chemical reactions that proceed with the absorption of light.

Photodynamic Therapy: A cancer treatment using a photosensitizing agent administered intravenously or topically which concentrates selectively in tumor cells, followed by exposure of the specific waves of light creating a photochemical destruction of the diseased tissue.

Photofrin: A light-activated drug used in photodynamic therapy.

Photomultiplier: An electronic sensing device used to detect electromagnetic energy of a wide range of wavelengths at very low levels, such as biophotons.

Photon: A particle of light, used as the basic unit and the force carrier electromagnetic radiation.

Photopheresis: A system in which blood is treated with photo-activable drugs which are then activated with ultraviolet light.

Photophysics: A field described as nonreactive relaxation processes, which include radiative (taking place with the emission of light) and nonradiative pathways.

Photoreceptor: A nerve ending, cell, or group of cells specialized to sense or receive light.

Photosensitizer: A light-absorbing substance that initiates a photochemical or photophysical reaction in another substance (molecule), and is not consumed in the reaction.

Physicochemical: Relating to both physical and chemical properties.

Pigments: A material that changes the color of reflected or transmitted light as the result of wavelength-selective absorption.

Pineal Gland: Small endocrine gland that produces a hormone that affects the modulation of wake/sleep patterns and seasonal functions.

Pituitary Gland: an endocrine gland located at the base of the brain and secretes hormones that regulate homeostasis.

Plasmid: A DNA molecule that is separate from, and can replicate independently of, the chromosomal DNA. Plasmids usually occur naturally in bacteria.

Platelet: An irregular, disc-shaped element in the blood that assists in blood clotting.

Platelet Aggregation: The clumping together of platelets in the blood.

Polychromatic: Used to describe light that exhibits more than one color or radiation of more than one wavelength.

Porphyrin: A group of organic compounds of which many occur in nature. The best-known porphyrins are; chlorophyll in plants, it converts light to energy and heme, the pigment in red blood cells.

Prion: An infectious agent composed of protein in a misfolded form.

Psoralen: A light sensitive compound containing chemicals that react with ultraviolet (UV) light.

PUVA: A therapy that uses Psoralen and UVA light to treat skin disorders.

Quantified: To prove empirically, verifying parameters.

Radiation: Describes a process in which energetic particles or waves travel through a medium or space.

Radachlorin: A light-activated drug used in photodynamic therapy.

Reflexotherapy: A form of therapy practiced as a treatment in alternative medicine in which the soles of the feet are massaged: designed to stimulate the blood supply and nerves and thus relieve tension.

Scotopic Vision: The vision of the eye under low light conditions.

Season Affected Disorder (SAD): A mood disorder characterized by mental depression, related to a certain season of the year, that occurs at the same time every year.

Sepsis: A Blood infection, it's a potentially serious medical condition characterized by a whole-body systemic inflammatory state.

Serotonin: A neurotransmitter primarily found in platelets and in the central nervous system of animals including humans. It is a well-known contributor to feelings of well-being.

Spasmus Nutans: A disorder affecting infants and young children. It involves rapid, uncontrolled eye movements, head bobbing, and occasionally, abnormal positioning of the neck.

Supermolecular: Term used to describe complexes of two or more molecules that are not covalently bonded. The term supermolecule is also used in biochemistry to describe complexes of biomolecules composed of multiple strands.

Sympathetic Nervous System: As part of the autonomic nervous system it aid in the control of internal organs.

Parasympathetic Nervous System: The part of the autonomic nervous system that inhibits or opposes the physiological effects of the sympathetic nervous system.

Temoporfin: A light-activated drug used in photodynamic therapy.

Thermodynamic: The effect of heat and time on different elements of matter, and or energy and their interrelationships that can be quantified.

Thoracic: An area of the spine that consists of the vertebrae located between the top of the neck and the top of the low back.

Thrombosis: The formation or presence of a blood clot in a blood vessel.

Toxoplasmotic: A parasitic disease. The main sources for this disease are cats and raw meat.

Transdermal: A route of administration wherein active ingredients or light are delivered on or through the skin.

Urogenital: Relating to both the urinary system, and to the interior and exterior genitalia.

Virus: A small infectious agent that can replicate only inside the living cells of organisms.

Viscosity: Quantification relative to the fluid's resistance to flow, its thickness or internal friction.

Watt: A measurement unit of current defined as one joule per second to quantify the rate of energy conversion.

White Blood Cells: Immune system's cells involved in defending the body against both infectious disease and foreign materials.

Honorary Dedication

Special Thanks to the visionaries that have changed light role on this planet. I graciously appreciate the brilliant minds that took the time to educate me, and now I'm passing it on the others, thank you.

Albert Einstein, Ph.D.	Eugene Barnett
Alexander Gurwitsch	Helen Irlen
Amy Cannon, Ph.D.	Henry Kaiser
Anita Saltmarche	Herodotus
Arun A. Darbar, D.D.S.	Hugo Bach
Aurelius Celsus	Jaimie Henderson, Ph.D.
Beverly Rubik, Ph.D.	James Carroll
Bill Levinson, Ph.D.	James Clerk Maxwell
Bob Distefano	Jane C. Wright, M.D.
Boris Zemelman, Ph.D.	Jean-François Grollier
Botond Roska	Joe S. Crane
Brian Hulbert	John Hearst, Ph.D.
Charles Townes	John Kennedy
Christoph Wilhelm Hufeland	John Ott (Honorary Doctorate)
Chuck Mooney	John Strisower
Chukuka Enwemeka, Ph.D.	Juanita Anders, Ph.D.
Darrin Brager, Ph.D.	K. Martinek
David Olszewski, E.E., I.E.	Katherine Creath, Ph.D.
Deborah Carroll	Kendric Smith, Ph.D.
Devon Perry	Kenneth Dillon, Ph.D.
Donald J. Stillwell	Kim Segal
Dr. Sidney Garfield	Krishna Shenoy, Ph.D.
Dr. Adam Landsman	Kurt Wedgely
Dr. Andre Mester	Len Saputo, M.D.
Dr. Auguste Rollier	Lynne McTaggart
Dr. Barbara Parry	Maha Sherifis
Dr. Bergein Overholt	Marco Bischof
Dr. Diane Mediguzzo	Margaret Abigail Cleaves
Dr. Dick Menzies	Max Planck
Dr. Fritz Hollwich	Melinda H. Connor, Ph.D.
Dr. George Brainard	Michael Hamblin, Ph.D.

Dr. George Miley	Michael T. Yen, M.D.
Dr. Gregory Raiport	Nathan S. Bryan, Ph.D.
Dr. Harry T. Whelan	Neils Finsen
Dr. Harry Wohlfarth	Osborne Eaves
Dr. Harvey Jay	Paul Bradley, D.D.S.
Dr. Helen Shaw	Paul E. Boccumini, Ph.D.
Dr. John Downing	Paul Weiner
Dr. José Rodriguez Delgado	Percy Hall
Dr. Joseph Meites	Herbert A. Pohl, Ph.D.
Dr. Karl Deisseroth	Pythagoras
Dr. Kenneth Mikkelsen	Richard Whyte, M.D.
Dr. Leonard Rudnick	Richard Wurtman, M.D.
Dr. Max Luscher	Rick Krupnick
Dr. McDaniel	Robert A. Weiss, M.D.
Dr. Richard Cremer	Robert Olney
Dr. Richard Edelson	Roblee Allen, M.D.
Dr. Shimon Rochkind	Ronald Hsu, M.D.
Dr. Thomas Dougherty	Ronald Waynant, Ph.D.
Dr. Tiina Karu	Roy G. Geronemus, M. D.
Dr. V.P. Kazmacheyev	S.V. Krakov
Dr. Virgil Hancock	Sandra Gollnick, Ph.D.
Dr. Wendell Krieg	Seymon Kirlian
Dr. William Campbell Douglass	Stacy Malkan
Dr. Zane Kime	Stephen Bown, M.D.
Edward Boyden	Stephen J. Fanning
Emma Ross	Steven Potter
Emmit S. Knott	Susana Q. Lima
Eugene Barnett	Suzanne L. Kilmer, M.D
Francisco Contreras, M.D.	Thomas DeMarse
Fred Kahn, M.D.	Thomas Dougherty, M.D.
Fritz-Albert Popp	Thomas Perez
Augustus J. Pleasanton	V. Berezin
Harvey Lui, M.D.	Veronica Stetson
Heeral R. Shah, M.D.	Walter Ude
Heinrich Hertz	Weijia Zhou, Ph.D.

Special Appreciation

Active Bacterial Core Surveillance
American Cancer Society
American Medical Association
American Medical Journal
American Society for Photobiology
Center for Disease Control
Central Texas Veterinary Specialty Hospital
Defense Advanced Research Projects Agency
Emerging Infections Programs
Federal Drug Administration
Finsen Institute
Health Medicine Institute
Hughes Research Laboratories
Johns Hopkins University School of Medicine
Kaiser Permanente
Infectious Diseases Society of America
International Institute of Biophysics
International Photodynamic Association
Institute of Human Biology
Irlen Institute
Lancet Medical Journal
Lawrence Berkeley National Laboratory
Livestrong.com
Marshall Space Flight Center
Medical Light Association
MIT Laboratories
National Association Space Aeronautics
National Center for Complementary and Alternative Medical
National Institute of Health
National Institute of Mental Health
National Research Institute of Physical Culture
New York Institute of Technology
Roswell Park Cancer Research Institute
Sarasota County Dental Society
Society of Cosmetic Chemists
State of the World Forum
The Center for Frontier Science
Transatlantic Task Force on Antibiotic Resistance
U.S. Department of Defense
U.S. Environmental Protection Agency
U.S. National Institute of Health
U.S. Navy
United States Government
World Health Organization

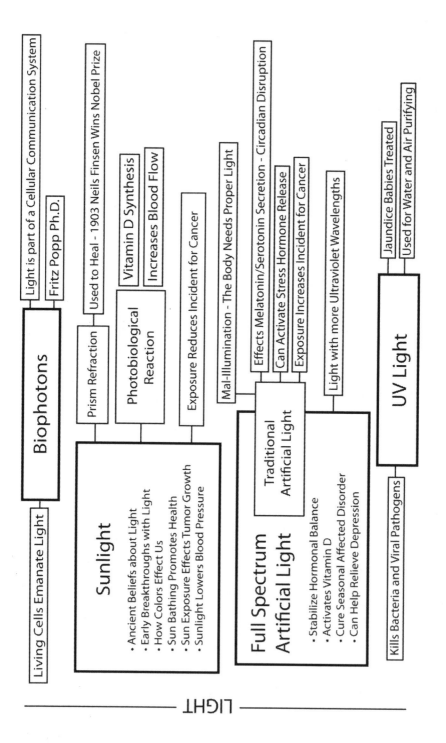

LIGHT

Biophotons

Light is part of a Cellular Communication System

Fritz Popp Ph.D.

Living Cells Emanate Light

Sunlight

Prism Refraction

Used to Heal - 1903 Neils Finsen Wins Nobel Prize

Photobiological Reaction

Vitamin D Synthesis

Increases Blood Flow

Exposure Reduces Incident for Cancer

· Ancient Beliefs about Light
· Early Breakthroughs with Light
· How Colors Effect Us
· Sun Bathing Promotes Health
· Sun Exposure Effects Tumor Growth
· Sunlight Lowers Blood Pressure

Full Spectrum Artificial Light

Traditional Artificial Light

Mal-Illumination – The Body Needs Proper Light

Effects Melatonin/Serotonin Secretion - Circadian Disruption

Can Activate Stress Hormone Release

Exposure Increases Incident for Cancer

Light with more Ultraviolet Wavelengths

· Stabilize Hormonal Balance
· Activates Vitamin D
· Cure Seasonal Affected Disorder
· Can Help Relieve Depression

UV Light

Jaundice Babies Treated

Used for Water and Air Purifying

Kills Bacteria and Viral Pathogens